Zigzagging

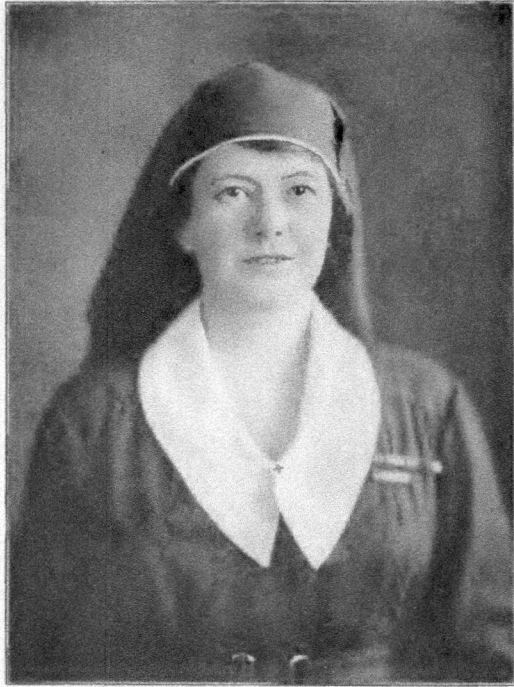

THE AUTHOR IN NURSE'S UNIFORM

Zigzagging

The Experiences of an American Red Cross Nurse
During the First World War

ILLUSTRATED

Isabel Anderson

(Mrs. Larz Anderson)

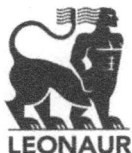

LEONAUR

Zigzagging
The Experiences of an American Red Cross Nurse During the First World War
By Isabel Anderson
(Mrs. Larz Anderson)

ILLUSTRATED

First published under the title
Zigzagging

Leonaur is an imprint of Oakpast Ltd

Copyright in this form © 2020 Oakpast Ltd

ISBN: 978-1-78282-944-7 (hardcover)
ISBN: 978-1-78282-945-4 (softcover)

http://www.leonaur.com

Publisher's Notes

Contents

DEDICATED
WITH SINCERE AFFECTION TO MY CO-WORKERS
IN CANTEEN AND HOSPITAL DURING
THE WAR, BOTH HERE AND
"OVERSEAS"

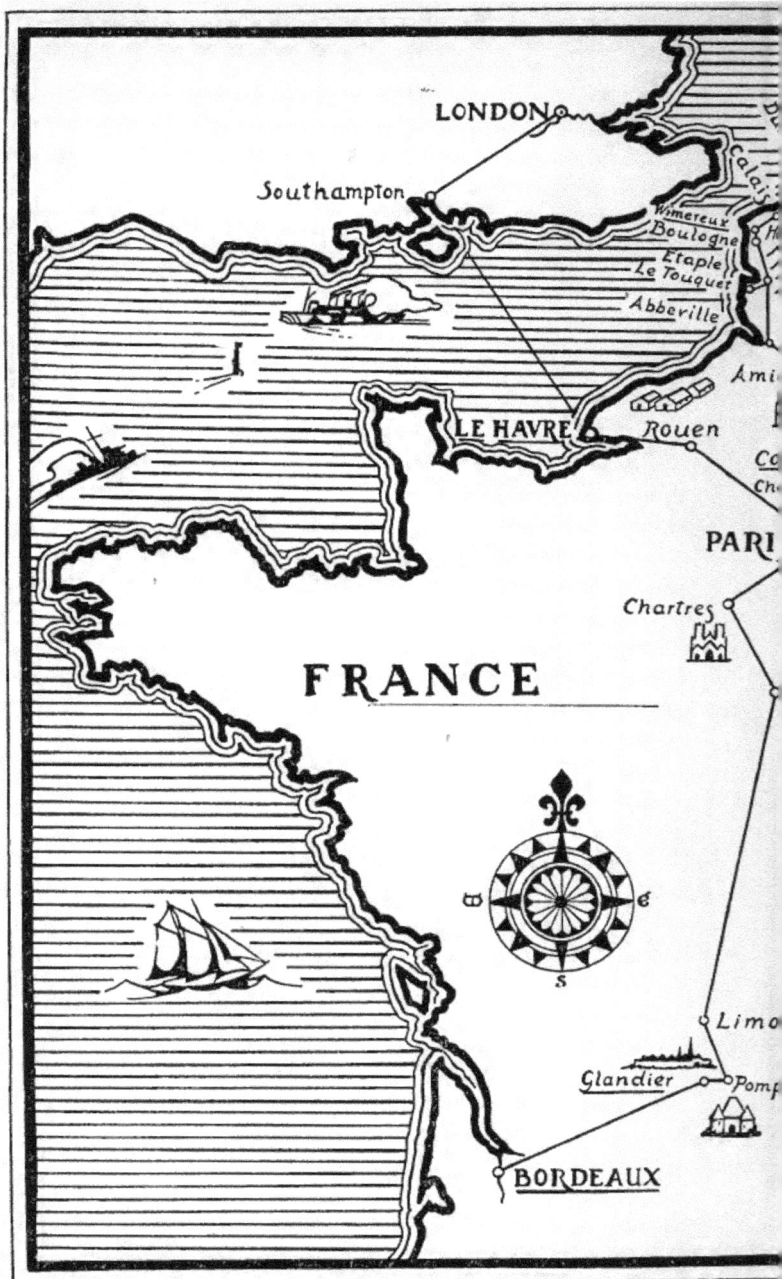

LONDON

Southampton

Calais

Wimereux
Boulogne

Etaple
Le Touquet

Abbeville

Ami

LE HAVRE

Rouen

Co
Ch

PARI

Chartres

FRANCE

W   E

S

Limo

Glandier   Pomp

BORDEAUX

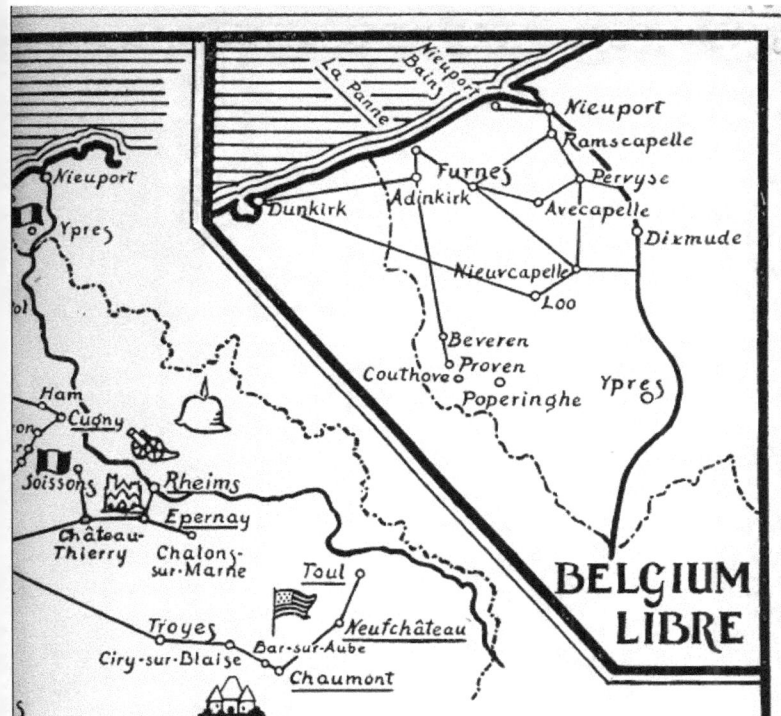

Nieuport
Nieuport Bains
La Panne
Ramscapelle
Furnes
Pervyse
Dunkirk
Adinkirk
Avecapelle
Dixmude
Nieucapelle
Loo
Beveren
Proven
Couthove
Ypres
Poperinghe

Nieuport
Ypres

Ham
Cugny
Soissons
Rheims
Epernay
Château-Thierry
Chalons-sur-Marne
Toul
Troyes
Neufchâteau
Ciry-sur-Blaise
Bar-sur-Aube
Chaumont

BELGIUM LIBRE

𝒟irections

———— Author's Route Line

———— Battle Line Mar. 20, 1918

—·—·—· Frontier

E. Crosby

Preface

Few people read prefaces nowadays, I know, but I am old-fashioned and one of the few who like to know in a word what I am to expect in a book. So, it is for those like myself that I am writing this.

To begin with, in these pages there is nothing but the truth as I saw it, and this is simply an account of my experiences, such as they were, written in the hope that they may help some other war workers. I was head of the canteen in Washington, but I was a private in Europe, so I know the trials and pleasures of both ranks, in this country and "over there." Workers must expect obstacles, and chief among these is the lack of opportunity for service in posts of danger, and for administrative work of any sort. But I will say more of that in a moment.

When I went to the publisher, he asked, "What new points have you got on the war?"

I answered, "I can tell you, from a woman's point of view, how it feels to be in the front-line trenches, and what an American woman's experiences are in an *auto-chir* or *triage* hospital moving with the French Army." (A distributing hospital six miles from the trenches, where operations are performed.)

"Anything else?"

"Well, I worked with an American Red Cross canteen in the army zone for a time, and assisted for several weeks in an operating-room with the Queen of Belgium, and among other things I had the good fortune to dine with General Pershing at headquarters at the American front."

"What do you plan to call the book?"

I offered several titles. I was tempted to joke and suggest *Female Feuds at the French Front*, but it seemed to me there were as many feuds among our war workers at home as abroad. Or *Female Fools at the Front*, for I had heard—I cannot vouch for the story—that an American worker in Paris cabled to headquarters in America:

Sending too many intelligent women—send some fools.

But this was too serious a moment to joke, and we compromised on *Zigzagging*.

Most of the women I saw, I am happy to say, were intelligent and good workers and went over from purely patriotic motives. Strong, level-headed women willing to do anything, go anywhere, and obey orders, are what is needed. Those who speak languages and are good mixers are especially useful, for to my mind one of our first duties on foreign soil is to get on amiably with our associates of other countries.

Women have a great field for organisation in America, but on the other side many women feel they are made the drudges of the war, because they are worked hard and kept mostly at the base, and even there they are not given many administrative duties. They are not allowed in or even very near the trenches as nurses, canteeners, or fighters, unless by special privilege, and in fact there are comparatively few opportunities given them anywhere in the army zone.

But turning to the histories, I find women have had their share in active warfare in the past, and I believe they are just as brave today (1918) if they are given a chance. There have been heroines of different kinds and of all nationalities and classes, peasants and queens, individual leaders and bands of fighters, from mythological days to the present time. Even in classical writers there are stories of the Amazons, who came from Ethiopia and overran Asia; of the women of Argos, who defended that city against the Spartans; of Boadicea, the British queen, who led in the slaughter of Roman legionaries.

There was Joan of Arc, the peasant girl whose story is too well known to repeat; and Queen Margaret of Anjou, wife of Henry VI of England, who during the Wars of the Roses rode at the head of the armies she raised, and at times commanded them. Isabella of Spain lived in a tent with her husband on the battlefields and also led her troops, as did Catherine the Great of Russia. At the siege of Haarlem, Ken-au Heselaer led three hundred women against the Spaniards. In the present war (1918) the Russian "Legion of Death" has become famous. (See also *Yashka* by Maria Botchkareva, commander of the 1st Russian Battalion of Death; Leonaur 2019.)

In olden days the Chinese and the native rulers of India had groups of women warriors. Perhaps the most noted fighting bands of African women were the eunuch-tended Congo and Dahomeyan Royal

Guards of the early part of the last century.

In our own Civil War, Señorita Loretta Velasquez enlisted under the name of Lieutenant Harry Buford and fought at Bull Run on the Confederate side. She was a Cuban who was married to a Southerner. Miss Beebe Bean, dressed like a man, joined the American Army in the Philippines and went soldiering for a year, in the Spanish War. Dr. James Barry, an Englishwoman, who also wore male attire, became inspector-general of army hospitals at Capetown in the Boer War, and was buried under her assumed name. (*Vide The Woman in Battle* by Loreta Janeta Velazquez; Leonaur 2010.)

There were many women fighters in the Balkan War, and one American woman, Ruth Farnam, holds the rank of sergeant in the Serbian army today, and has been several times decorated, while Sergeant-Major Flora Sandes, an English woman in the same army, has received the highest order a Serbian soldier can win. (*Vide Sergeants Ruth and Flora* by Ruth S. Farnam & Flora Sandes; Leonaur 2014.)

In the great army of those who have shown their bravery as nurses stand out two never-to-be-forgotten names, Florence Nightingale and Edith Cavell. (*Vide Nurse Edith Cavell* by William Thomson Hill; Leonaur 2011.)

Women today may prefer to be canteeners or nurses rather than fighters, but they do want a chance to work at the front, where they can be of the most service, not coddled in comparative safety at the bases. After all, hasn't a woman just as much right to die for her country as a man?

Brookline
August 8, 1918

CHAPTER 1

Zigzagging

The Red Cross sent out a demand for fifty canteen workers for overseas duty. Of course, those already in canteen service were preferred, and I felt it my duty to go. Such a hurry to start! I had an interview with Miss Marshall at the national headquarters in Washington, and she told me to report in New York the next morning and to sail in ten days, if possible. Telegrams, packing, weepy goodbyes, midnight train—all in one twenty-four hours. My friends either did not approve of my going or were most enthusiastic, but all snivelled, until I decided I would not tell anyone else, but just slip off.

Thousands of soldiers were going through Washington at this time, and the Red Cross canteen of which I had charge was more than busy, and short-handed, too. I went flying here and there, giving instructions to the corps, visiting Red Cross rooms, and signing papers. Miss Marshall presented me with a circular of information for canteen workers overseas, which I studied on the train. (See Appendix.)

During my short stay in New York City I bought warm clothing, matches, sugar, candles, soap, and other things that I was told I might need in France, but which I afterward found I could buy just as well over there—though, to be sure, they were more expensive; then I went to New Hampshire to see my mother for a few days. Back again to New York, where passports were obtained, photographs taken, and letters received from the Red Cross officials. These last were quite unnecessary, for, on arriving at headquarters in Paris, I could find nobody who wanted to read them. Though they were from high officials of the Red Cross here, everybody was too busy to look at them. By the Red Cross regulations workers were allowed to take only a steamer trunk and a dress-suit case, and it was a masterpiece of packing that stowed away all the necessary articles in so small a space. No fur coats were required, I heard, which was a great mistake, for they are really very much needed.

My husband and I were very sad at the prospect of a separation but we both had war work, it was war-time, and we felt patriotic. At last, after he had made all my arrangements for traveling, he left me in my stateroom on board the *Espagne*. During the evening the owner of the French line, M. Perrin de la Touche, and M. Franklin-Bouillon, then Minister of the Foreign Office, came on board. Everybody cheered. The gangplank was pulled up, and our ship glided out into the blackness of the night, leaving behind the twinkling lights of the great city of New York, while the enormous statue of Liberty with her flaming torch lighted the heavens. It all seemed a strange dream. Was it possible that I was quite alone and on my way to France in war-time?

It was impossible to find my own chair on deck, so I finally took an empty one. A man soon came groping along and sat down nearby. He proved to be an Italian on his way to Venice to buy laces. My next chair neighbour was an Englishman who had been an interpreter for the British Army in Belgium. Before we landed, my acquaintances proved to be of many sorts. I talked with M. Franklin-Bouillon about conditions in France and with M. de la Touche about U-boats, and with Captain Girot about the army, as well as with Mr. Perkins and several others of the Red Cross and the Y.M.C.A.

The first night I went to bed in a real nightgown, but finding it too much work to dress In the morning, after that I slept in my clothes, as it was necessary to do for months at the front. This voyage was not different from others except in the darkness of the passageways and the complete blackness of the decks. I could not see one thing. It was positively spooky, and it made me feel more and more my absolute aloneness in the world.

The next morning, we were in the midst of a wild storm and the boat plunged through the spray of high waves. I managed, however, to go down to all my meals, and found myself at a small table with a nurse who had been in France during the war, and a man on his way to Portugal to buy cork from the large cork-oak groves of that country.

On looking about, I found most of the Y.M.C.A. workers exercised every day on deck, and listened to lessons in French and lectures on the sex question. The Red Cross men were rather sporty and smart-looking in their uniforms, while the Red Cross nurses reminded me of school teachers. There was a very pretty girl in khaki who caused much amusement, as it was said she planned to drive a motor, with bath-house attached, from place to place for the convenience of aviators. Hundreds of Armenians at this time were going back to fight, and every day I watched them in their tight clothes and fur caps as they were drilling in the steerage.

The voyage was smooth and warm and peaceful. We might have been on the Pacific until we reached the danger zone. Then it became colder and fog settled upon us. Our ship began to zigzag. We tried on our frog-like rubber life-saving suits, and all assembled on deck before the boats. In the staterooms we had found papers telling us which life boat or raft to take in case of disaster. Mine was No. 7. The people for that boat were far from pleasing. I did not feel like drowning with them.

Six of us women slept side by side in a corner on deck, with our passports and money upon us and our life-belts beside us—it was very warm below—and we told stories and giggled like school girls. Even if the bed was hard, it was fun to watch people prowling round in the darkness.

There was superb phosphorescence one night. Never even in the China Sea have I seen it so brilliant; the sensation was as if we were sailing over the moon or a ball of glowing crystal—it was unearthly and mysterious.

A day or so before we arrived, we saw floating wreckage on the water, and the *Espagne* shot once at a supposed mine and three times at a submarine or an overturned boat in the distance. The passengers were all agog! People seized their glasses and rushed to the upper deck. We changed our course and zigzagged even more, for the supposedly overturned boat seemed to be suspiciously moving with us.

Our shots fell short of it, and it did not return the compliment. It was said, however, we were chased by a submarine that evening. As a rule, they appear at dawn in smooth weather.

The last night on board we had an auction, and people paid huge sums for trash. We sighted two French torpedo-destroyers, and then steamed up the river, past the welcome green fields and pretty houses to Bordeaux. At the docks were great French liners, and German prisoners at work, and American soldiers who gave us a rousing cheer. As the U-boats were working then in flotillas, the French ships were putting on longer-range guns, which accounted for so many being at the docks. It was also said they would no longer carry the Swiss mail.

In other words, this line had probably been quite safe up to that time, as by it the Germans got mail through Switzerland. It was even rumoured that spies travelled by these ships, for not one had so far been torpedoed.

Our luggage was brought up, and we stood in line before tables on the deck and showed our passports. There were few porters to be found on landing, and I all but carried my trunk on my back myself. Up and down the gangplank three times I went, and after much difficulty, with the help of some friends, finally got my small bags, camera, typewriter, etc., to the station. But by that time, I was in a state of perspiration and wrath.

Having several hours in Bordeaux, some of the workers visited an American base hospital, a Harvard unit, made up of doctors from Boston. It was well organised in a beautiful old school building in a park five miles out of town. The nurses lived in barracks and had cot beds in big rooms like the patients. There were, however, few patients at that time.

After seeing the lovely cathedral, four of us dined at quite an amusing restaurant, where there were plenty of good things to eat. There seemed to be many men in the streets and endless little dogs, showing, I felt, that there was more food than I expected in France. One would think with the food shortage more of these cur dogs should be shot, as has been done in England. The only sign of war I saw in Bordeaux was that the conductors on the trams were girls, and the town seemed full of American soldiers, who gathered about us and asked for news of home.

The taxi man who took us to the train that night drove at such speed that it was a wonder we were not killed. Another canteen worker shared the same compartment with me. It was too dark to see anything along the way, but we heard there were few signs of war, if any, in this part of the country.

On arriving in Paris, in the early morning, we were very fortunate in getting two men porters—a rare circumstance, for most of the porters in Paris are women. We were put into a car and were greeted by a Red Cross man with, "Will you go to a *pension*, two in a room, including meals, twelve *francs* a day; or Hotel Regina with single room, fourteen *francs?*" Four of us "old girls" decided to go to the hotel; the younger members of the party went to a pension with Mrs. G., who was in charge of the canteen contingent.

The driver, like the taxi man of the night before, went at such speed that we first collided with a motor and then with the corner, and all our bags flew out and sprang open. Sponge bags and underclothes rolled and fluttered over the street.

I drew the very worst room engaged by the Red Cross at the hotel. It was in the attic. It was dirty. You could see only the sky and a little piece of a roof. There was one red blanket, and the room was too small for even a chair. Yet I really became attached to my attic, and began to think the red blanket cheerful. I enjoyed watching the aeroplanes in the sky. At a desk which I made for myself out of my traveling bags and by the light of two candles stuck into old bottles, these notes of my life in France as a canteen worker were begun.

Paris, I found in many respects the same wonderful, gay, charming city that it had always been—with the same crowded boulevards, full of movement and life; the same broad Tuileries, the same Champs-Élysées and Bois; but now filled with smart-looking English and American officers.

The Paris of old, with the delicious little breakfasts, the *cafés complets*, the flaky white bread smelling so fresh, the pat of butter looking so cool and white, and an incense rising from the boiled milk that could nowhere else be obtained, was not quite the same. The bread was dark brown, the milk condensed, and there was no butter at all. The one thing I missed more than anything else after a night journey was a hot bath. They gave hot water only on Saturdays.

We reported at the Red Cross building, a big structure that had once been a palace and then a clubhouse, whose rooms with red carpets, high ceilings and crystal chandeliers, although not exactly the customary style of office, made a very good headquarters. Here we found Mrs. Vanderbilt, who was in charge of the canteen workers, and were given more rules. We visited three police stations, signed endless papers, and wrote over and over again how old we were, and who our mothers and fathers and grandfathers were, and where we were born, and what our occupation was, etc., etc. (See Appendix.)

Our canteen uniform for outdoor wear, a grey jacket and skirt, bought in New York, was somewhat changed. We were told to have French horizon-blue collars and cuffs put on, which we liked. The uniform has since been changed again; now it has U.S.A. on it. Big blue aprons with white collar and cuffs and white *coiffes* to wear when working in the canteen had to be ordered, as they were different from the canteen uniforms worn in America; so, with all the new requirements we were kept busy.

There seemed to be thousands of Red Cross men dashing in and out of headquarters. All were so busy that they did not have time to speak even to a friend. Major Murphy was then at the head, and Mr.

Perkins the second in command. Major Murphy has now resigned, and Major Perkins is at the head of all American Red Cross work in Europe. There have been many changes, and the organisation is steadily improving. The men are all in uniform and have military rank, such as major or captain. Most of the younger men have now gone into the army.

The contrasts in war-time are especially funny. While I was living in my attic and traipsing round in the Métro for two *sous*, with other canteen workers, I was having tea with our American ambassadress, Mrs. Sharp, with a princess, and a Minister of State.

One delightful Sunday was spent in the country at Madame de la Touche's pretty villa. An artist, a writer, and an aviator took me out in a motor. M. de la Touche and his wife were most hospitable and, in our honour, made American cocktails—which were very bad, but which we appreciated, nevertheless. We wandered about the picturesque farm and the well-kept park. They were dear, kind people, and I enjoyed my day.

Since the war broke out, a host of organisations have been formed and carried on by Americans residing in France for the relief of sufferers by the war, but most of them have now been absorbed by the Red Cross. One of the best known is the American Ambulance at Neuilly, which Mrs. Vanderbilt took me to see. It certainly is well run, and the Boston ward is one of the largest. There I saw the huge magnet that draws out shrapnel, and the Carrel treatment with Dakin solution, which is dropped from a bottle hung at the bedpost into a tube and from that upon the wound.

It was wonderful to see how this simple antiseptic solution, which is at bottom nothing more than common chloride of lime, healed gangrenous sores, raw wounds upon which the new cuticle would not form, or deep-seated inflammation of the bone. Before this treatment was discovered, so many infections—such as erysipelas, lock-jaw, gangrene—followed surgical operations that, even if the patient recovered from a compound fracture, it was almost always necessary to amputate the limb as blood poisoning generally set in. But Dr. Carrel proved, by persistent research, that skilful treatment would sterilise even a septic wound. On Dr. Carrel's staff were Dr. Dakin, of New York City, and Dr. Daufresne, of Paris. Dr. Dakin's work was to free the chloride of lime from an irritating alkali and then, with the help of Dr. Daufresne, to find a way to prepare it in absolute purity and of just the right strength.

GRAND QUARTIER AMÉRICAIN DU CORPS EXPEDITIONNAIRE
HEADQUARTERS AMERICAN EXPEDITIONARY FORCES

Paris, 6 *Octobre 1917*

De la part de l'ADJUDANT GÉNÉRAL au Major G. M. P. MURPHY
From : Adjutant General To : Major G. M. P. Murphy.

Armée Américaine, Commissaire de la Croix-Rouge Américaine pour l'Europe.
American Army, Commissioner of the American Red Cross for Europe.

SUJET : *Autorisation de visiter dans la Zone des armées*
SUBJECT : Authorization to visit the Zone

Le COMMANDANT EN CHEF du Corps Expéditionnaire Américain autorise les représentants
The COMMANDER IN CHIEF, American Expeditionary Forces, authorizes the following representatives
suivants (militarisés) de la Croix-Rouge Américaine :
(militarized) of the American Red Cross :

Mrs Isabel Hamilton Andersen
(aide pour cantine)

a se rendre aux endroits suivants : *Epernay*
to proceed to the following points

où ils auront à rendre compte aux autorités *militaires* du travail spécifié ci-dessous :
where they will report to the authorities for the work as hereunder specified
travail à la cantine

Une fois ce travail terminé ils devront retourner à leur poste ordinaire.
Upon completion of this work they will return to their proper station.

Mode de locomotion *chemin de fer*
Mode of travel

Cette autorisation est donnée avec la permission du Grand Quartier Général Français, étant
This authorization is given under permission of the French General Headquarters with the understanding
bien entendu que ces représentants de la Croix Rouge Américaine (militarisés) sont soumis à toutes les
that these representatives of the American Red Cross (militarized) are subject to all the orders and
ordonnances et à tous les règlements publiés pour l'information et la conduite des soldats et auxiliaires
regulations published for the information and guidance of soldiers and camp followers of the American
des Armées Françaises et Américaines.
and

Par Ordre du Major Général Pershing :
By command of Major General Pershing :

BENJAMIN ALVORD,
Adjudant Général
Adjutant General

Officiel :
Official :

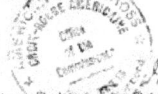

Major du Corps de réserve des États-Unis,
Major of the U. S. Reserve Corps,
Commissaire de la Croix-Rouge Américaine pour l'Europe
Commissioner of the American Red Cross for Europe

PASS TO WORK IN CANTEEN IN ARMY ZONE

Another efficient co-worker with Dr. Carrel was Miss Grace Cassette, who for two years superintended the surgical dressing-room of the American hospital at Neuilly. She found the usual orthopaedic appliances were not what were needed for fractures received in battle, and so she invented new ones, which held the limbs firmly, so that the wounds could be drained and amputation avoided. One surgeon said of their work:

"With Dr. Carrel's solution and Miss Cassette's splints we can save many limbs that would otherwise have to be amputated."

Among her patients was a man who because of two broken vertebrae had worn a plaster cast for months, so heavy that he could not walk. She made an aluminum corset for him and padded it well inside, and, in Miss Cassette's words, "the first day he wore it he walked about normally, as happy as a child." The French Government has made her a *Chevalier* of the Legion of Honour.

While in Paris waiting for orders, I was able to do a little work in Dr. Blake's hospital, now called American Red Cross Military Hospital No. 2. This was built by a famous French surgeon, and was considered the most magnificent hospital of its kind in Europe. Dr. Blake has been in France ever since the outbreak of the war, and the institution soon became famous for the fine surgery performed there. It was here I first saw badly wounded soldiers, and dressings done for those whose limbs had been amputated. Dr. Blake's appliances for fractures are also very noted.

There were two canteens in the Care du Nord, where I likewise helped a little. Both were in the cellar, and needless to say, they were dark and cheerless. The English soldiers, who are paid fifty cents a day, get a good hot dinner, but pay for it; the Americans and Colonials, who receive a dollar a day, also pay for their meals. But French and Belgian soldiers, who get only five *sous*, have a meal free and also a bed, if they have no other place to sleep. During the spring drive I worked for a few days in the dispensary, taking care of sick refugees.

At last orders came for me to go to Épernay, on the Marne. Leaving my steamer trunk with friends, I packed my bags in the little attic room, paid my bill, and started early one morning. I found three other canteeners on the same train, but they were strangers to me.

Our journey was through the valley of the Marne, and we had hardly more than passed beyond the suburbs of Paris when we approached places whose names thrilled us with recollections of the drive in 1914. Between Lagny and Meaux the British Expeditionary

Force retreated over the river, followed by von Kluck in that reckless diagonal march to the southeast that exposed his flank to attack by the Anglo-French forces. All along the Marne, from Changis through Château-Thierry and Mézy, the hosts under von Kluck and von Bülow poured across. The same section of the river was hurriedly repassed by the Germans in their flight northward, with the British "Contemptibles," better called "Indomitables," close upon their rear. (*Vide Contemptible* by Casualty (an "Old Contemptible"'s recollections); Leonaur, 2012.)

Northwest of Meaux was the scene of the fierce fighting between General Maunoury's soldiers and von Kluck's rear-guard. Through five days of burning heat, beginning September 5, the French kept up the battle in the face of overwhelming forces which the Germans recalled from beyond the Marne. On the 9th they faced almost certain disaster. They woke on the morning of the 10th to find that the enemy had disappeared. Why? Because fifty miles to the eastward General Foch had made his wonderful dash through the gap between the marshes of Saint-Gond and La Fère Champenoise, and, supported by all those other incomparable Frenchmen, had changed the situation from impending defeat to victory.

Twice before in history, the fate of Europe had been determined on the soil of France—once at Chalone, when Attila and his Huns were routed, and again at Tours, when the armies of the Saracens were driven back—but a still greater battle had just been fought in this valley. The very soul of civilization had been saved, and the world breathed more freely.

The Battle of the Marne was fought not far from the railroad, but too far away for us to see the white crosses marking the heroes' graves. I little thought that before these notes were given to the public another even more titanic struggle would be under way in the same quiet valley. But we saw no sign of war, the river flowed peacefully in its fertile basin bordered by lines of trees. And at last we arrived at Épernay.

CHAPTER 2

A Canteen on the Marne

Les Français, en guerre,
Sont de vrais poilus—
(Choeur) Poilus!
La Patrie est frère
De ses chers Poilus,
(Choeur) Poilus!
Le Boche rccule,
Sachant bien qu'ils sont
Costauds comma Hercule
Et comme Samson.

There was no one to meet us at Épernay, and not a porter or a cab in sight. What were we to do with our bags? They were too heavy for us to think of carrying ourselves. Across the square from the station many blue-coats were hovering round a shack where a couple of English women were giving out coffee. But they were too far away to see our predicament. At last we found a handcart, and hired a boy to push it, and set out to follow our property on foot.

The grey town looked as if it were in the bottom of a teacup, with hills all about. Although it is comparatively new, with the handsome villas of champagne kings and a *Grand' Place* in the centre of the town, it had its picturesque corners, too—the canal, where the women were doing their washing in primitive fashion, and the bombed houses, for the Boches seemed to enjoy visiting the peaceful little town.

Not far from the station and almost hidden by the trees of a small park, stood a low barrack, painted green, with French and American flags flying side by side. This was the Cantine des Deux Drapeaux, where I was to work. The French furnished the land and the barrack

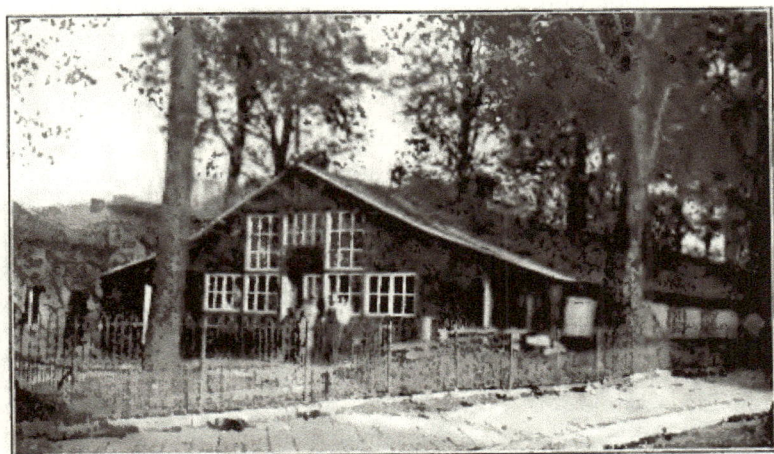

THE CANTEEN AT ÉPERNAY

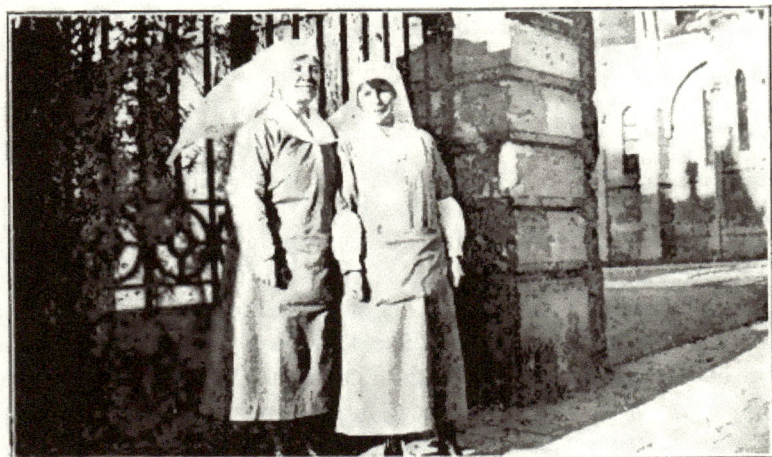

MISS LANSING AND MISS MITCHELL IN CANTEEN COSTUME

and the fuel, while the Americans paid for food and service.

We did not stop to look inside, but went on past the church and climbed up the narrow, winding, cobble-stoned street till we came to 9, rue des Minimes. This was a good-looking stone house with an iron fence and a little yard with a weeping-willow tree in front of it. Here we were to live. Miss Lansing, sister of our Secretary of State, received us, and later the directress appeared and gave me a nice room. As I entered, I saw signs of war in a grey gas-mask hanging in the hall, and a raincoat camouflaged like an autumn leaf.

After luncheon at the hotel, I got into my blue apron with white collar and cuffs, and my flowing *coiffe*, and set off to work, for my first shift began at one o'clock and lasted till seven in the evening.

On the outside the Canteen of the Two Flags looked dark and dreary enough. But inside it was brightened by some orange-coloured camouflage grass hanging from the roof, and we soon made it quite gay with pretty posters, and curtains at the windows, and yellow lamps suspended from beams. At night, when the lamps were lighted and the room was full of *poilus*, sitting at tables, their blue uniforms veiled in the smoke of their cigarettes, it made a fascinating picture.

The canteens run by women are situated at railway centres, where the largest possible number of fighting men can be accommodated. Those nearer the trenches are run by men. For these, all that is really essential is a room with a counter over which the drinks are served to the passing soldiers, a small storeroom for keeping the materials, and a stove or rolling kitchen where the water can be boiled. But our canteen was well equipped and served regular meals. Men going home on leave thus have a chance to clean up and rest and get a good meal, and they go home much more contented and cheerful as a result. In this way the canteens do a great deal to keep up the morale of the troops.

In our canteen, adjoining the big hall we had a kitchen, an officers' room, a first-aid department, and a small writing-room, as well as a wine room—the last run by soldiers. There were two openings in the wall between the big hall and the kitchen, through which the food was served. When I first went on duty, I served chocolate and coffee—the coffee free, but chocolate four *sous*—salad, cheese, nuts, and confitures at one of these windows; later I took the other one, where I passed out the *repas* of soup and *ragoût* or tripe. In addition, we had to ask a deposit of fifty *centimes* for the spoons, knives, and forks, which was troublesome, but it was made necessary by their rapid disappearance. The *repas* was served from ten until two, in the middle of the day, and later from four until nine. But soup and other things were ready all day and all night.

There were sixteen American women in our canteen, who served three or four on a shift, while twelve French women took turns in the kitchen, cooking and washing dishes. During the twenty-four hours we fed from one to two thousand men.

★★★★★★

At one of the canteens the Red Cross served two hundred and sixty-five meals in two and a half hours, an average of about one meal every thirty-four seconds. At another, coffee was served at the rate of one cup every two seconds over a period of several hours.

★★★★★★

Signs were put up outside the windows where the soldiers could see them: *"Repas, 75 centimes"*; *"Soupe, 15"*; *"Legumes, 15"*; *"Viande, 50"*; *"Salade, 30"*; *"Confitures, 25"*; *"Fromage, 30"*; *"Oeufs, 50."* In the kitchen other signs showed the proportions to be used in cooking, such as, "Three bowls of powdered coffee, one bowl of chicory," etc. (The *poilus* wanted the chicory.) These measures were later changed to grams.

The women at the *caisse* or desk sold tickets for the various articles of food. The *repas* tickets ran about four hundred a day, and bread tickets averaged about the same, while chocolate and coffee tickets sometimes went as high as eight hundred. At the end of the month there was very little loss, showing that the restaurant was under particularly good management, for we were supposed to sell under cost. (See Appendix.)

Miss Lansing and I started a store there in the canteen, buying our goods from the French "cooperative." The things which the *poilus* liked best were tobacco, which was sixty *centimes* a package and very bad, cigarettes, at fifty-five, and electric torches, three *francs*, eighty. We also had a few canned goods for them to take on the march. It was run only in the evening, when the cooperative and the shops in the town were closed, in order not to conflict with them.

On Sundays the *poilus* received magazines and cigarettes free, as a present from the workers, and at Christmas the Red Cross gave each soldier a free dinner and a surprise bag; the English women had a concert for them in the evening. (See Appendix.)

Across the street from the canteen was a *"Maison du Soldat,"* where some of the men slept on hospital stretchers. The English women had

27

a *salle de lecture* there, larger than ours, but only open a short time each morning and evening. Their "*Goutte de Café*" near the station served free *jus* (slang for coffee) but merely at certain hours—while we were cleaning the canteen in the morning, for instance, or when extra troop trains were going through—so we worked well together.

The rest of this chapter is taken directly from my journal, written on the spot during the autumn:—

"I cannot say enough in favour of the *poilus*. They are brave, cheery, polite, and grateful, too. The more I see of them the better I like them, and the finer I think they are. So many have asked me to be their *marraine* that I feel as if I were godmother to the whole French Army. They love to write letters. (See Appendix.) Of course, they often sing in the canteen, and here is one of the songs they sing to their *marraine*.—

Ma Marraine! Chanson de Poilu, par Griff

E - tant en perm' tout der - nier'- ment, J'suis
al - lé voir ben gen - ti - ment, ma mar - rai - ne!
Cel' qui m'en - voy' des p'tits pa - quets, Pour
la pre - mier' fois, j'la voy - ais, Ma mar - rai - ne!

"As they do not know exactly what kind of people we are here at the canteen, they ask us many questions. Are we paid? How old are we? Could we find them a wife, or marry them after the war? Since the red-*fezzed Zouaves* have gone, the *poilus* in blue are much better behaved. But the *Zouaves* are great fighters, and I admire them.

"Our regulations (see Appendix), specify that we must always answer their questions pleasantly and never argue with them.

"Last evening, we had an artist in the canteen, a soldier who made pictures and threw them across the counter to us. On one he wrote, 'Hip, hip, hurrah for the American ladies!'

"We certainly have had some amusing experiences. A *poilu* came in today and asked for a bowl of hot water. He set it on the counter and took his glass eye out and washed it. Another did the same with his false teeth, while still a third took advantage of the opportunity to shave.

"We see but few wounded, although I have tied up a good many hands that had old wounds or new cuts. The other night two men got fighting in the canteen with knives, and one had his arm badly slashed. Another time a *poilu* picked up a bottle and threw it at his opponent's head, yelling, 'This *brancardier* did not bring in my wounded comrade!' There have been several fist fights, too. But nearly always, even after *pinard* (slang for wine), if one says, 'No discussion in the canteen, please—ladies are present,' they will stop.

"The heat from the stove in the kitchen and the cold, smoky air from the counter in the canteen, added to the moisture from the dripping roof, have given us all what is known as the canteen cough.

"I am comparatively comfortable in my room at the house on rue des Minimes. It has two windows with blue curtains, a good bed, and an *armoire*, and two small tables and a rug which I bought myself. It is so cold I go to bed between the blankets with my clothes on and a hot-water bottle. In the morning I wash with the water from this bottle, which is warmer than that in the pitcher. Then I breakfast in my room, on George Washington coffee and crackers, or sometimes malted milk and a piece of chocolate. The other meals are served here in the house; the food is good. Our expenses are nine *francs* a day, and for that sum we live very well.

"As twelve of us women live together in one house, I feel as if I were in a grown-up boarding-school, or a convent. For afternoon tea, I walk out to the corner and buy chestnuts from an old woman. The days slip by with the work and a letter and my walk, besides washing my hands and gargling my throat at intervals, for the canteen is full of germs and smells.

"A canteen worker who crossed on the steamer with me has arrived, looking like a wreck. It is a month since I saw her last, and she has been working twelve hours a day at Issoudun for the American aviators, cooking for those who were ill.

★★★★★★

The original pioneer band of Red Cross workers who came to France have been added to until today (1918) there are one hundred times as many in the organisation. In order to care for this Red Cross army, the Medical Division has taken the matter up, and now all the workers receive medical, dental, and hospital care free of charge. Thirty beds for their use have been established in the American Hospital in Paris and seventy in the American Red Cross Hospital at Neuilly. These are also at the disposal of the Y.M.C.A. and the Y.W.C.A.

★★★★★★

"I am writing now by the light of two guttering candles, with my toes in the gasoline stove. The great buzz of a fleet of *avions* comes to my ears, and I run to the window to look out. By the light of the full moon they look like wicked darning needles off for their prey. How the stars do twinkle these winter nights! They are so big that I often take them for *avions* with lights. Sometimes they are. One quite alone flew down near the spires of the cathedral, darting in and out of the clouds like a soul that had lost its way.

"The Germans have machines now which can go over the line so quietly that the French cannot detect them, and so of course they are sometimes unable to warn the inhabitants. People are leaving town for the week of the full moon, as bombs are always dropped then.

"Sometimes I look out at night and see ghostlike regiments marching silently past. Again, I am wakened by the clatter of hoofs on the cobble stones. Opening my window and turning on my flashlight, I see a mounted troop turning the corner of the street, with cannon, and kitchen wagons drawn by horses, lumbering along behind. When I walk up on the hill in the evening, I can distinctly hear the roar of the big guns pounding Rheims.

"English aviators and American ambulance boys visit the canteen as well as the *poilus*, and our American troops, our marines and engineers are not far away.

"Frenchmen of all ages up to forty-six, and from all parts of France, are fighting side by side. They say it is better to mix the troops from the north and south, as those from the north fight better. Soldiers coming from the Swiss border who have German names are given French ones for the war, because the Government realises that the Boches will not spare a French captive with a German name.

"There are several big military hospitals here in Épernay, where both soldiers and civilians are cared for. The Convent of Notre Dame in the *Grand' Place* has been turned into one especially for head wounds, which includes those who have been blinded. Some of the face cases are so disfigured that they are frightful beyond any words to describe. But the patients seem astonishingly cheerful. The other day, when an attack had been going on between Rheims and Châlons, I counted twenty-five ambulances passing through the town. I hear a number of Americans have been killed in Alsace-Lorraine. They were holding a reserve trench and had too much light in it, poor fellows!

"German flying machines go over constantly in the daytime to observe and take photos. As soon as they are seen, the anti-aircraft guns are heard and the little white puffs of smoke appear in the sky. Like a child, I never get tired of rushing to the door to look at them. One day when we were out for a walk, and the shrapnel fell all about us, we crawled under a wagon for shelter.

"What an excitement in the canteen the nights we are bombed, when the whistle goes off, warning us that the Boches are coming! Our orders are that all the soldiers must leave for the *abri*, and ourselves as well, but this is difficult to manage. The men are used to danger, and are comfortable and warm where they are, and they don't want to leave. Moreover, some of them are always asleep on the floor. We don't like to run away ourselves and leave our *caisse* unprotected for fear it may be robbed. Once I stayed there with one other woman all through the middle of the night, entirely in the dark, with at least eight more or less drunken *poilus* for company, but they all behaved well.

"Another night we stood in the *abri* until nearly morning—canteeners, cooks, and a dozen *poilus*. The shelter which we used was a sort of deep, covered trench dug in the churchyard, narrow and zigzagging, and lighted only by our little electric flashes.

"Épernay at night is a city of utter blackness. I don't understand why I am not afraid to go home from the canteen quite alone at midnight. I hear the clatter of approaching feet on the cobble-stones, or a motor feeling its way without a light, and perhaps see a quick flicker from a flashlight, but that is all. Even on Sunday nights, when people are out by the hundreds, walking up and down the main street in the darkness, there is no disturbance. The soldiers are not noisy or badly behaved, and one can go anywhere and seldom be so much as spoken to.

"I did feel a trifle nervous the other night, I must confess, when I walked two miles through a strange part of the town with a bottle of champagne under my arm. It was a present for a birthday party, and I was afraid some soldiers might see the bottle and take it away from me, but nothing happened.

"It all feels like another world, and I have to pinch myself sometimes to make sure I know where I am and what my name is.

"We hear there are night attacks constantly at the front, near Rheims, and that much gas is used. The fighting is more active than last winter. Many soldiers seem to be going to Italy, and there are numerous changes among the officers here. It is said the English made a clever surprise attack and captured many guns not far from us. We really have little news, however. Telegrams are posted outside the station, but sometimes days go by without our seeing a newspaper. From what we do hear, it appears as if the situation were very bad, with Russia going back on us and a hundred thousand or more Italians taken prisoners.

"What artistic little pictures one can see in this country! Against a gay wall stands a tall, jet-black soldier with bright blue uniform and red cap, holding the bridle of a superb bay Arab stallion. A little bent old woman with a big sunbonnet and heavy boots trudges along the muddy road, carrying a primitive hoe at least a century old, and the fields behind her form a background.

"In the entrance to the cathedral stands a little statue of Joan of Arc, and always at her feet are fresh, pretty flowers. In the church one is sure to find soldiers at their prayers, and women in mourning. The grey arches, the stained glass in the windows, the lighted candles, the music, and the silence when there is no music, give one a feeling of sadness and homesickness that is hard to express.

"Today two of us took a *diligence* drawn by an old white horse that trotted us out to a small village nearby. Our fellow passengers were a soldier and his sweetheart—he called her his *belle-soeur*, though—and two women from the regions invaded. Such sad stories as I hear! It is hard to realise that they are true—but they are.

"As the moon is full again this week, many people go from Épernay to this village to sleep, because they believe the Boches will not find it worthwhile to bomb so small a place. Of those who remain in town, many sleep in their *abris*.

"Several American officers, among them General Scott, dined with us at the inn. As we were crossing the *Place* a Boche airplane flew over and star lights appeared in the sky. Then the antiaircraft guns from the town began firing. We stood on the corner and watched, hoping they would bring it down, but nothing further happened, so we went on to the hotel.

"We have had a luncheon for General Gouraud and his staff, including the Comte de Chandon, who is one of the big champagne people here. He sent us some beautiful chrysanthemums, and also a more prosaic gift, though no less appreciated, of fish and potatoes. General Gouraud, who is one of the two most talked-of generals in the French Army—the other being Petain—has only one arm, and is

32

a stern-looking man, blond with cold, steel-blue eyes. A shell landed near him once, and he was blown into the air, striking against a tree which tore his arm so badly that it had to be amputated.

"The other night we dined with Comte de Chandon, whose *château* with its courtyard and sunken garden was half closed. The Germans had lived there for five days while on their march toward Paris in 1914. Although they had drunk much champagne, they fortunately did little damage, and when they went back through Épernay, they were in too much of a hurry to stop for further destruction. Later on, their aviators returned and threw a lot of bombs on the place, some even flying so low that they fired into the windows. The *comte* took us through vast champagne *caves*, the cellars where thousands of bottles of wine were stored.

"Yesterday morning I awoke out of a dead sleep to hear the church bells ringing a tune that they played over and over again. The music had a haunting sadness that rang in my ear, and in spite of the cold I got out of bed and wrote down the notes. It was All Souls' Day, and the bells were chiming for the dead.

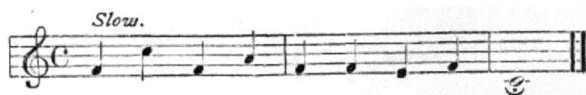

"From the telegrams at the post-office door, and from what we hear in the canteen, as well as from the movement of troops through the town and the number of flying machines over our heads, it seems that fighting is active all about us. Some English girls have appeared, driving ambulances. There is a rumour that a good many British have been taken prisoners at Cambrai.

"I shall never forget what a picture the *Grand' Place* was early one morning, when everything was sprinkled with glistening snow. There were shivering *poilus*, and tired horses, and great camouflaged guns, and cook stoves, and *camions*, all huddled together resting for a moment before they pushed on.

"Last night the booming of the guns was so loud, coming with the wind like the roar of the ocean, that I felt sure the Germans were moving upon us.

"Some strange characters turn up at the canteen. A crazy Arab worked all day bringing in dishes to the window. It was a great help, but he would take no recompense. Another man worked like a beaver for us for three days, and said it made him feel at home. He was a *poilu*

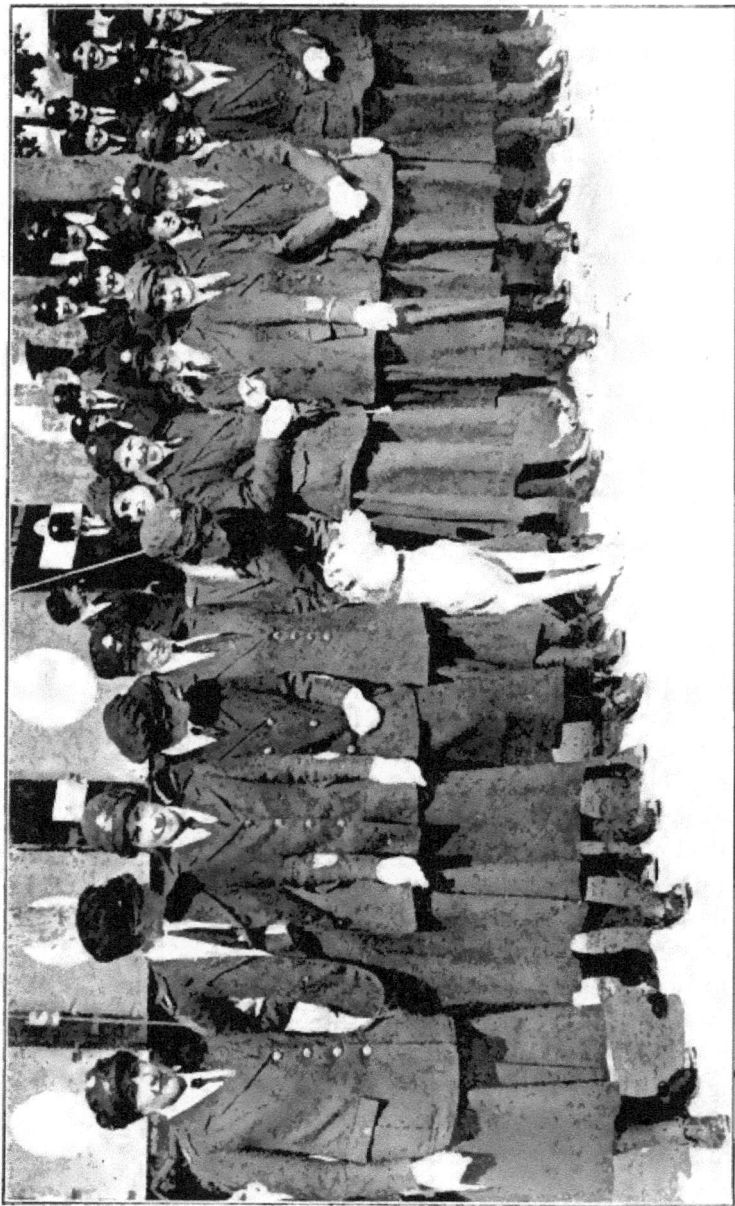

AMBULANCE-DRIVERS ON THE BRITISH WESTERN FRONT

just out of hospital, who had run a restaurant before the war. His wife was a nurse, and he wept as he showed me her picture.

"A bent old refugee appeared. She had no money and no place to sleep, so we let her stay in the kitchen and peel potatoes. Later, when I asked for her, one of the kitchen girls told me she had gone. '*Grand'mère* had *bêtes*' (cooties), she explained. All the women in the kitchen have sad stories. Either their husbands are prisoners, or they themselves have suffered in the invaded districts. (See Appendix.) One girl who lived in the region overrun by the Germans said the behaviour of the soldiers depended entirely upon the officers.

"Not long ago I walked to a neighbouring village where some Colonial troops were stationed and saw some of the much talked-of 'seventy-fives,' the rapid repeating guns that the Germans do not seem able to copy, as they are fired by a combination of glycerine and compressed air. Hundreds of shaggy horses, many of which had been in the war since the beginning, and frisky, kicking mules, were tied in the open. The *poilus* do not like our American horses, which they say are too wild—coming over the sea makes them *fous*, they declare. They prefer their own, or English or Arabian.

"Another day I had leave to go to Châlons-sur-Marne. My *carnet rouge* had been left downstairs, and I did not find it, so I came near losing my train in consequence. When it was given to me by a kind friend who finally discovered it, there were only ten minutes left to catch the train, without allowing any time for breakfast. I couldn't even wash my face and hands, because we had had visitors the night before and they had used the water and towel in my room.

"Then, after all that hurry and excitement, the train was late, and I had to sit for a long time in the cold waiting-room before it came. There was nothing to be seen outside, because all the windows looking out on the station platform had been painted, to prevent one's seeing the troops that pass.

"The traveling public consisted of officers and ladies in crape. Along the way were the usual villages nestling among vineyards, and the familiar straight roads lined with poplars. The only signs of war were a pontoon bridge and a regiment *en route*.

"Châlons is now a great military centre, and the station was bristling with *poilus* as the train drew in. I waded through the mud to the American canteen, which was not so quaint and primitive as ours, but by far the most complete and elaborate one on the front. The big hall, whose walls were frescoed in *nouveau art*, was square and high-posted,

35

and had many tables and a long counter, much like a station restaurant at home except that there were no doughnuts and pies. I got a cup of black coffee and a piece of cheese, and was about to indulge in something that looked like baked beans, when I discovered a friend who carried me off for a walk by the river.

"Our walk took us over a fine old bridge, the only one the Germans left across the Marne. In the little gardens along the road there were roses still in bloom, though somewhat nipped by the cold.

"After a look at two beautiful churches, begun in the twelfth century, where much of the fine old glass has been broken, I took my *carnet rouge* to the police for examination. I ended the day by taking tea with some of my cousins who were canteen workers there, and then returned in the dark to Épernay in time to do my night 'keep.'"(See Appendix.)

CHAPTER 3

In the Trenches at Rheims

We were amused at hearing of an American ambulance boy who got into Rheims with a chewing-gum label as a pass, but there was so much unnecessary gadding about, that the American Red Cross and the French became very strict in regard to permits. By great good luck I got one, however, as I had a letter from the French Minister of War.

I had to go alone from Épernay in the motor *de voyage*—and a real adventure it was. Looking like a *poilu* in a raincoat with bulging pockets and big boots, with grey gas-mask and bag slung over my shoulder, I started out. Of course, there were difficulties in getting a ticket and a seat, but at last a place was found where I could open the flap and look out occasionally. The great lumbering green thing began to buzz, and we were off.

After showing our passes, we slowly trundled on, over the rolling hills with vineyards where sticks were piled in little bundles like beehives. As the bus approached Rheims, we saw signs that the road had often been shelled, and on the side toward the Boche trenches was a camouflage screen twelve feet high, made of netting with wisps of brown raffia. Later a grey camouflage veil appeared, put up in the same manner along the road, with an occasional opening to look through. Although we were not far off, it was so misty that one could not detect the line of the German trenches.

Information was difficult to get in Épernay, and before reaching Rheims, I made two alarming discoveries—no hotel was open there, and the motor did not return that evening. I was wondering what to do, and trying to make some inquiries, when a jolly woman sitting near me in the motor offered to have her boy show me about and find me a place to stay.

As we drew into Rheims it seemed like a city stricken with plague, for it was quite deserted. Hardly anyone was in the streets, not even soldiers—they were in the trenches. There were a few women in the market-place arranging vegetables, and that was about all,

I helped the kindly woman carry her huge package home. She lived in a second-rate wine-shop not far from the cathedral. The little shop contained four dogs, two children, and an old man, as well as a woman who kept the place in her absence—she was just returning from Paris where she had been to see someone in a hospital.

Her husband, it seemed, was a prisoner in Germany, and a *blessé* as well. She cooked me some eggs and gave me some green-grey oysters, which I ate, thinking that as I had been inoculated for typhoid, they might not hurt me. To crown her kindness, she offered to put me up for the night if I could not find anywhere else to go. Leaving my bag with her and telling her that I might return to sleep there, I started out with the boy as guide.

The Place Royale was surrounded by houses all cracked and open to the weather, showing the disordered rooms inside with tumbled beds, just as the people had deserted them in a hurry. A basin of blood stood on the floor in one house. What a smell of decay! A city of wounds, weeping, and bleeding.

The *curé* of Épernay —who has lately been killed by a bomb in front of his own door—gave me a letter to the cardinal, so we entered the courtyard of *Monseigneur's* fine residence near the cathedral. A sister met me there and showed me into a small reception-room, where presently the vicar general appeared. Unfortunately, Cardinal Luçon, (see Appendix), was in Paris for a few days, but the vicar said he would take me inside the cathedral, and he gave me a letter to the *commandant*.

This poem, written by an American ambulance man, might very well apply to the wonderful Cardinal of Rheims,

> *The Priest*
> *I saw him first in the Rue Royale*
> *And was struck by his kind old face—*
> *With his sable robe and golden cross,*
> *And air of delicate grace.*
> *He greeted the poorest girl of the streets*
> *And the greatest dame of the land,*
> *With the same sad smile and a gentle nod*
> *And a friendly wave of the hand.*

I thought of the grand old cardinals
Who lived in the long ago;
Whose stories are part of the stories of France—
And their lives in their great châteaux.

And then came the fight for Malmaison,
I saw my priest again,
With gas-mask and blue steel helmet
Standing alone in the rain.
He stood at a crowded cross-roads
In a mud-bespattered gown.
The shells were falling about him
As the wounded came straggling down.

His own chasseurs and poilus,
Arabs and Senegalese,
For each a smile and a cigarette.
And a cheery "Bonne chance, mon fils."
And a wave to me as I passed him
(I was driving an ambulance)
And the thought was always before me
There stands the Spirit of France!
Simple and brave and courageous,
Gentle and débonnaire,—
The cause of the Church is surely safe,
With men like him Out There!

Stephen Pell
Somewhere in France

The Hotel Lion d'Or, where my husband and I had lunched some years before, was still standing, but closed and much battered. In front of it was a huge *obus* hole with a drain trickling through. Nearby stood the exquisite statue of Joan of Arc, untouched except that the uplifted sword in her hand was slightly bent.

There is no need that I should add another to the many descriptions of the Cathedral of Notre Dame at Rheims. Before the war it brooded over the Champagne like a great sphinx, dominating the modern town of manufacture and trade as centuries ago it dominated this coronation town of kings.

The most gorgeous of French cathedrals, dating from the twelfth century, no more magnificent stage could have been devised for the royal pageant that here opened every reign but one from 1173 to the time of Napoleon. It was here, too, that Joan of Arc enjoyed the triumph of her career. After delivering Rheims from the English she herself gave the keys of the city to Charles VII.

To me the lace-like shell of the cathedral seemed more beautiful in its distress and desolation than it had in the days of its splendour. It was like someone lying in the coffin, all the imperfections of life stripped away, nothing but the beauty of peace and the spirit of God left. One did not notice the stupid head of the donkey thrust out from the walls, and the grinning gargoyles.

The interior was bare indeed. The wonderful thirteenth-century windows were shattered by the first bombardment, as we all know, but the fine old tapestries that draped the walls, the statues that filled countless niches throughout the church, the Sainte Ampoule with its holy oil brought from heaven by a dove for the baptism of Clovis, and the other priceless relics, have all been removed to Paris.

I was given as souvenirs some bits of yellow-green thirteen-century glass, and a piece of a Boche *obus* which had fallen within the church. As I was leaving, a motor appeared with some newspaper men, the Ambassador of Siam, a Red Cross representative, and a couple of women.

The little boy led me on through more abandoned streets, among tottering buildings, through alleys and fields, till we came to the *Bureau de Place*, which was in a comparatively safe place. It seemed like a haunted house with its weedy, neglected garden. I presented my letter of introduction and was received by the *commandant*, who said that in the morning he would give me his motor to see the town. When he asked where he should find me, the truth had to be told that, alas! I did not know where to sleep, but had left my bag at a little shop. He then took me back to the shop, where we got my bag, and left me in the care of a Madame Lambert.

Madame Lambert, assisted by another woman, also kept a sort of small restaurant. We three dined together, and they told me their story—their husbands were both at the front, and their children had been sent off for safety. They said that only a few doors away six women had been killed but a short time before—blown to pieces so there was nothing to bury. They had been able to get plenty of food from the beginning of the war, but prices were high. Nevertheless, they gave me three meals, as good as I could get on Fifth Avenue, with white wine, and rum in the tea, and only charged me twelve *francs*.

No one is supposed to be in the streets of Rheims after nine o'clock at night. As a rule, these women never went out in the evening, but they said they would go out with me to see the cathedral by moonlight. We had not gone far, though, when we heard a bang and a whizz which sounded just over our heads; they proved to be Boche gas shells, fortunately not near enough to do us any harm. There was no smell of gas, but some of the new gases have no odour.

There were many different noises during the night, but the guns sounded no louder than a Fourth-of-July evening with rockets and fire crackers—not half so lively, as a Wild West show. Dogs barked and motors rumbled, and once I heard a scream of agony from some wounded man going by in an ambulance.

My room was not exactly warm, for there was no glass in the windows, only cloth. I went to sleep under a feather bed, completely dressed, with my gas-mask hanging nearby. Madame Lambert and I could have slept in the *abri*, but we preferred taking our chances in the rooms one flight up. Several times in the night I thought I smelled gas, but there were so many smells it was easy to make mistakes. I did not put on my mask, anyway, and felt none the worse in the morning.

Soon after breakfast a captain came for me in a motor and we started off to see the town and trenches. The Hôtel de Ville was a complete wreck. The Roman mosaic left on the walls was unguarded. The rain dripped through the cracks. A handsome chandelier lay in pieces on the floor. A huge deserted hospital was riddled with *obus* holes, and its tangled gardens with old bronze ornaments of curling black snakes—the emblem of medicine—were, sadly dilapidated.

As we neared the trenches, which make a half-circle round the city, there was hardly a complete house left standing. My escort told me there were passages under the city that the soldiers used when the bombing was heavy, but this was a quiet, overcast day, so we drove along the streets on the surface. In the last houses, on the outskirts, before the fields were reached, there were deserted communicating trenches with holes in the walls for guns. In one of these trenches I found a pansy blooming; to me it was the symbol of some brave soul, some *poilu* who had died for his country.

The black hole of a passageway, dropping apparently into the bowels of the earth, proved to contain the trench quarters of the *brancardiers*, where there were bunks built into the earthy walls. Here the *blessés* were given first aid, then were carried out and put in ambulances and taken on to a hospital seven miles away—often to Épernay, if they had bad head wounds or were blinded.

Each regiment has its own kitchens. I saw one in the cellar of a demolished house and it looked very primitive and inadequate. Great *marmites* of soup and meat were carried by hand down flights of steps and underground into the trenches.

I have no expression of admiration too great for the *poilus* who have to live and sleep and fight in the dark, earthy passages of this hell. The captain said we were less than half a mile from the Boche lines.

Altogether too soon the exciting morning came to an end. I went back to Madame Lambert, who cooked me some eggs, and was all ready to start for Épernay when I was told that it was impossible to get a seat in the motor bus, as everything had been taken for three days! The pass gave me only two days, and my work was waiting for that night at Épernay. I had visions of going in an ambulance or a *camion*, or even of walking the thirty kilometres on foot. But at the last minute someone gave out, so there was a seat after all.

My fellow travellers were of many sorts, and their talk was very interesting. A wounded soldier was much upset over the Russian situation. Another did not seem to care much about the French Government. One criticised America—said she had been too long in coming into the war. Another got into a great state of excitement because his pass was questioned in a small town along the way. I learned that the government and the military did not agree any too well, and that in the spring before there had been revolts in the French Army.

Épernay at last, and my marvellous trip was over. Doubtless there had been some danger in it, but I would not have missed it for anything, as it gave me my first vivid picture of the devastation wrought by the war, and my first glimpse of the trenches.

That night at twelve o'clock I cleaned twenty-four tables, and when I came on duty next morning at seven, with the moon still shining, I cleaned the whole twenty-four again. The woman at the desk was not feeling well and could not help, and the third on the shift was scrubbing the kitchen and arranging things in the *cave*.

My own room was in dreadful disorder; friends had been in late the night before and sat on the bed, on the floor, on the slop pail; my things were scattered everywhere. I was feeling tired and cross with everything in the world, when—a telegram came summoning me to Paris.

Packing up my belongings, I hired a handcart to take them to the station, made the usual call on the police, and said farewell to the *commandant*. On the way to the station I stopped at the canteen to say goodbye. The cooks wept hysterically, especially old Marie, the dish-washer, who was a dear. My fellow canteeners appeared sorry to have me go, and indeed I regretted leaving them and Épernay.

Down the black street I went, quite alone in the middle of the night and in a pouring rain. The train was so late that I curled up on a bench in the waiting-room with the *poilus* and slept till three in the morning. At the critical moment, just as the train arrived, my flashlight gave out; but I managed to follow some officers into the train. The first car we entered appeared to be filled. In the second car I asked the person ahead of me if he would kindly tell me whether he saw an empty seat, as I had no light. He found one for me at last, and I wedged myself into the corner of a compartment with seven officers. It was hermetically sealed, and I felt as if in a Turkish bath. It was very dark and very silent, and I was so exhausted that I slept till the light of morning waked me.

At the station in Paris it took a long time to find my luggage, and a longer time to find a taxi. After signing at the American Bureau and the Red Cross, I went to three hotels, trying to get in. None of them had any room, but finally the Ritz let me have a huge pallor and gave me a nice suite the next day.

This was the end of my experience in the canteen, and the beginning of my *permission* in Paris, before I began working in the hospitals at the front for the French and Belgians.

CHAPTER 4

Auto-Chir No. 7

On arriving in Europe, I had quickly seen that the only interesting place to work was as near the trenches as possible. About Christmastime I had a chance to be transferred from the canteen to the hospital department to move with the Third French Army in the Auto-Chir No. 7.

★★★★★★

No. 7, a mobile hospital practically on wheels and ready to move at any time on short notice, attached to a French evacuating hospital of fifteen hundred beds near the front.

★★★★★★

I was very glad to join Mrs. Daly's unit of American women, which was then working in this barrack hospital at Cugny, about seven miles from the trenches and not far from Ham and Noyon.

The next things to be arranged were my passes and papers, which had to be signed by the French officials, and took about ten days. In the meantime, I bought my hospital uniform. The French nurses wear white dresses and veils, and we were to have the same, so my big blue canteen aprons had to be discarded. For street wear we had navy-blue serge dresses with a blue veil having a French cockade on the side, and a blue cape with brass buttons and the red cross.

My Christmas was typical for a worker in Paris. I lunched with Americans, dined with French, and all the afternoon distributed presents in the hospitals—flowers, postcards, and cigarettes, and beads for the men to make chains, and materials for them to do embroidery as they lay in bed. They did enjoy their treat of champagne and cake, and the concerts which were held in the wards.

One day a French captain took me to see the decorations bestowed at Les Invalides. We entered the huge hall, which was all misty with smoke, and saw the brave soldiers in their horizon-blue uniforms marching to gay music in the centre, while the galleries were crowded with onlookers. It was a marvellous spectacle. It hardly seemed real, but like a great war picture. But then, much I saw overseas did not seem real. It was hard to tell what was real and what unreal, so many things were unbelievable.

There were several lines of soldiers drawn up in the hall, some lame, some bandaged, some in wheel chairs. The general went down the line, and standing before each one made his citation with remarks, tapped the soldier on the shoulder with his sword, kissed him on both cheeks, and then pinned the decoration on the hero's breast. It was very impressive as he went from one to another in the dead silence. After this the band piped up cheerfully and the veterans withdrew to one side, where *les infirmières* were grouped with their *blessés*. The relatives of the dead heroes were then lined up—there were widows in long crape veils with little children clinging to their skirts, and weeping, grey-haired fathers and mothers. When the general came to them you could hear sobs all over the hall, and indeed my eyes were wet as well. This was the end, and we passed out of the sad grey-blue picture into the bright sunlight of the gay streets, where the snow was glistening.

Speaking of decorations, the *Croix de Guerre*, I found, is generally given to the *grands blessés* and dead, which perhaps is the right method, but every man who goes over the top in this war is a hero, and there are many marked cases of bravery in which a man is not wounded and consequently never receives a medal.

With other canteeners, I was asked to dinner by some American officers, and I was interested to see their quarters, which proved to be a charming apartment. Apparently, it had belonged to a lady of taste, and the satin-lined rooms and *boudoirs* with Chinese porcelains and rare prints must have made a contrast not only to their homes in America, but to the trenches which they afterward inhabited.

A well-known old deputy took us to the "*Chambre*" one day and put us in the President's box, as it was not occupied. Unfortunately, it was not an exciting moment, but the old Frenchman told us many interesting things. It appeared that he had visited the *Kaiser* every year and was with him a short time before the war broke out. He felt that the *Kaiser* himself did not want the war at this time, but that the crown prince and his followers, with the aid of the empress had forced him into it. I also heard this confirmed later by a Belgian of high standing.

The day for my departure arrived at last. As usual the train left at dawn. One of the canteen workers saw me off at the station, for which I was duly grateful. My hospital days were about to begin.

Traveling north, past quaint little towns, we reached Compiègne, where I changed cars and met some fellow nurses. From there on, our way led through the country where the Boches had been in 1914, not far from Coucy, where they had absolutely levelled to the earth the finest specimen of *donjon* in Europe, past old trenches and barbed wire to Noyon. All this part of France, which has now been for the second time invaded, is for that reason of great interest.

Noyon is an ancient town—with the remains of a wall built by the Romans—where Charlemagne was crowned, Hugh Capet elected king, and Calvin born. To come down to the present war, when the British Expeditionary Force made that wonderful retreat after Mons and Le Cateau, with exhausted bodies but undaunted spirits, they had their first halt along the Oise, at Noyon and near-by towns.

At Noyon we found a truck driven by a Scotch girl with the name of Richardson; she had been driving an ambulance during the Serbian retreat and in Roumania and Salonica as well. Our other *camion* driver was Irish, and she, too, had received all kinds of medals, and had driven an ambulance from Archangel to the Black Sea. These two girls lived in a big, double-lined tent, made of green canvas with isinglass windows, which stood next to our barracks. They generally cooked their own meals, but occasionally for a change came in to eat with us or went to the village of Cugny, where there was a small British canteen which served coffee for the *poilus* and showed them moving pictures.

Well, we packed the *camion* full of luggage, with the help of a soldier, jumped aboard ourselves, and were off along a straight road about eight kilometres to the hospital Auto-Chir No. 7. Through several villages we went that had been slightly bombarded, where soldiers were billeted, with signs outside the houses, such as "Horn. 3," "Horn. 6," showing how many men they contained.

The hospital buildings looked like a cross between racing-stables on a track and a Japanese Shinto temple, with a slight resemblance to a logging camp. In other words, many long, low, unpainted barracks, with small cloth windows. We had two of these barracks for the American nurses; one of them contained the dining-room and kitchen and the servants' quarters, as well as our Red Cross hospital materials; the other was our dormitory.

On entering this one, all I could see was a dark, smoky corridor with a stove at each end and lined on either side with white sheets.

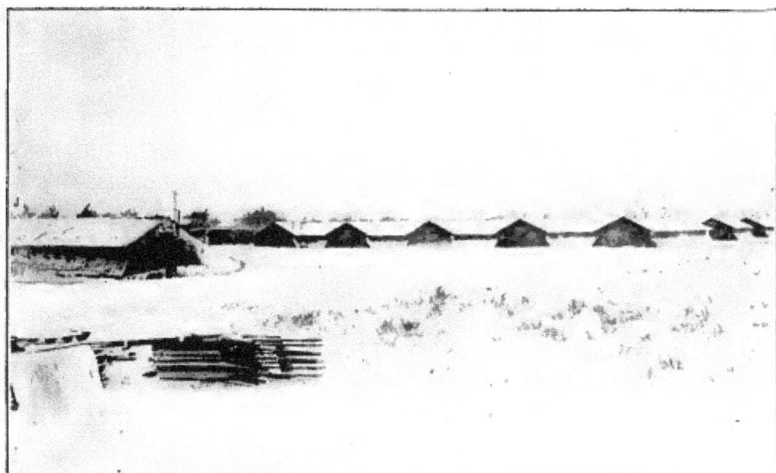

CUGNY HOSPITAL: GENERAL VIEW

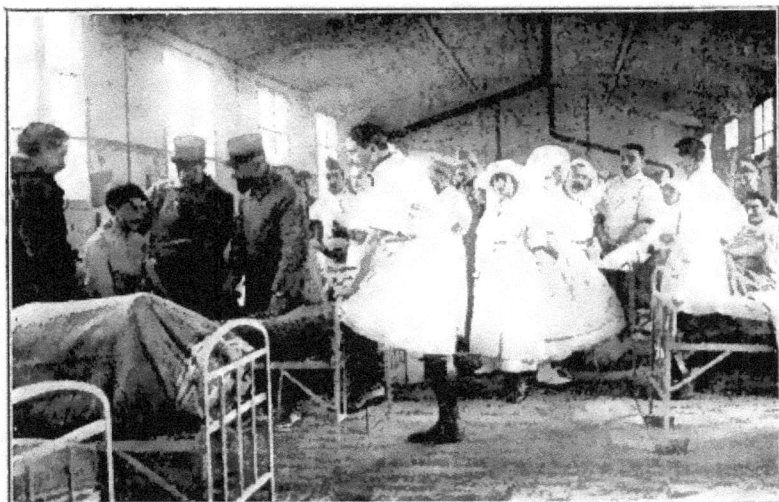

CUGNY HOSPITAL: INTERIOR OF ONE OF THE WARDS

I pulled back a sheet and found myself in the tiny enclosure which was to be my home for some time to come. It contained a cot bed, a packing-box with a pitcher upon it—and that was all. Later, however, it was made homelike with some pink chintz, and two more boxes, which I called my dressing-table and desk, and two blankets on the floor for rugs, which made me quite comfortable. And can you believe it, I had an electric light over the bed!

Conspicuous among the barracks was the *triage*, or hospital receiving-room, marked by a Red Cross flag outside to show ambulance drivers where to bring the wounded. The *triage* contained a room with stretchers and blankets where the wounded were received, and two *salles d'attente* where they waited their turn for the X-ray and operating-rooms.

An adjoining room contained a stove, and benches for the priest orderlies, who took down histories and recorded the time and place where wounds were received. A table with materials for dressings, and an alcohol lamp, which was constantly burning for sterilizing syringes and needles, were the only other furnishings.

The *infirmière* stationed here gives hypodermics, also gargling and nasal treatment preparatory to operations, supplies the hot-water bag and nightshirt, reinforces the dressings hurriedly put on at the *poste de secours* on the front line, besides helping bathe and undress the men, as there are only two orderlies for this work. The poverty of France after four years of war is shown by the reluctance of orderlies to cut uniforms. Rather than sacrifice the clothes they often pull them off the *blessé* and cause him needless pain.

A nurse is supposed to accompany every man on the stretcher to keep him from falling off while the *brancardiers* carry him. Many *blessés* who enter are delirious, but when conscious they are very brave and grateful for every attention.

During an attack the lack of surgeons to operate sometimes keeps men waiting all night upon a stretcher. When this happens, the single *infirmière* on duty alone must watch all the waiting wounded and stop their haemorrhages. It is she, likewise, who prepares the list of the most urgent cases to be looked after.

The first sounds we heard on waking in the early morning were those of the soldier making the fires, and then the tramp of Germaine, the girl-of-all-work. Her clothes were ill-fitting and she herself lopsided, her feet and hands enormous; she resembled an ungainly colt which hadn't learned to handle itself. Her movements were rapid but heavy, and as she ambled down the corridor the whole building shook. When Germaine was first heard, from all directions came calls behind curtains—"*L'eau chaude!*" "*Est-ce que le café est prêt?*" She was always cheerful, hard-working and obliging, but at intervals from her thick, drooping lips, her deep, raucous voice bellowed, "*Quelle horreur!*"

Our excellent chef was a wounded soldier, and he had two women from the village to help him. The girl who was supposed to wait on the table didn't wait at all, but sat by the stove conversing, and we generally went to the stove ourselves when we wanted something really hot. In the 1914 drive her father and two brothers were carried off by the Boches, and she had never heard from them since. They took a hundred people from her village back to Germany, mostly girls about fifteen years old. Occasionally their mothers were allowed to go with them. Our waitress said while the Germans were here the people worked for them without pay, and they would have starved if it had not been for the American relief under Hoover.

But to return to Germaine, in the early morning at last there would come a yell, "*Café prêt!*" I would slip out of bed and into a *Jaeger* wrapper and Indian slippers, and put a lump of my sugar—that came from America—into a tin cup, and make my way to the end of the barrack, where I found some canned milk and a hunk of bread. Then I would go to the stove in the corridor and pour out the coffee and toast my bread, which generally fell on the floor and got full of ashes, but I would put a little nasty butter or *oleo* on it, and really enjoy it.

My white uniform would be quickly slipped on, and at eight o'clock I was on duty. Drawing on rubber boots and carrying low white shoes, we crossed to another barrack through mud and snow. I was first put into *salle* 1, for the *grands blessés*, with an excellent nurse, and I can tell you she worked me! For two solid weeks I stayed until late at night, with only an hour off at noon.

Mrs. Daly's unit took care of only the surgical cases. The hospital had, of course, a large department for the *malades*, into which the gassed patients were put. There were operating-rooms and *pansements*, or dressing-rooms, with long, dark, draughty corridors, out of which open the different *salles*.

As this was a distributing hospital, the worst cases, of course, were left here in the *auto-chir*. The *petits blessés* were sent to other hospitals farther back, but during the winter a good many patients were kept in this one, for it was said, as the staff of nurses and surgeons was to be there, it was more economical to keep some of the wounded rather

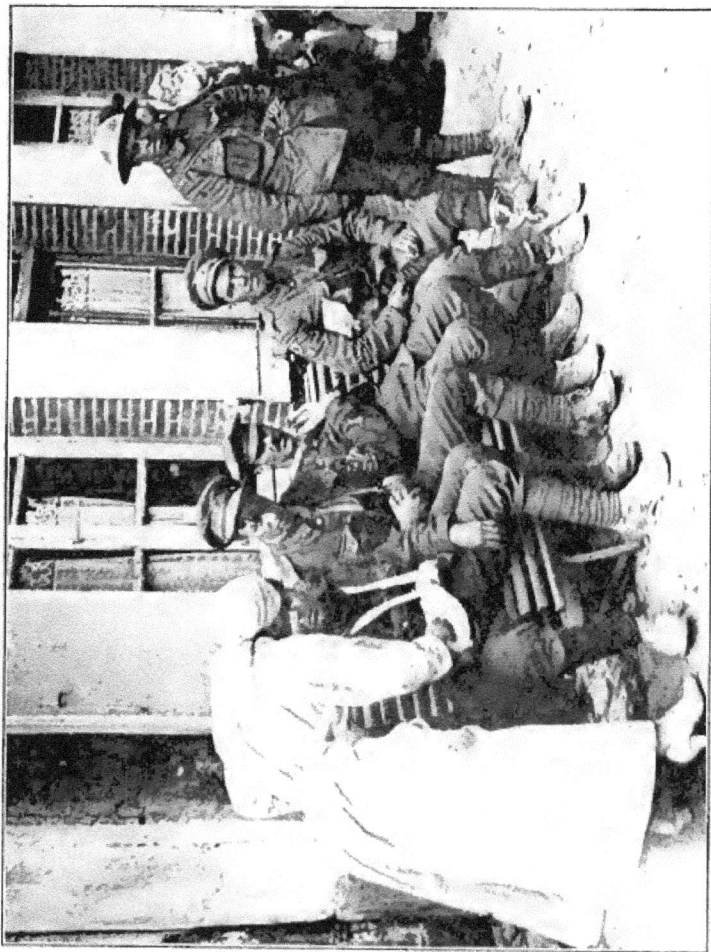

A FRENCH NURSE ATTENDING TO WOUNDED TOMMIES OUTSIDE A SMALL VIL-
LAGE ESTAMINET WHICH HAS BEEN CONVERTED INTO A TEMPORARY HOSPITAL

than move them when they got better.

In our *salle* we had only from fifteen to twenty wounded—it was called a dull moment!—but they were all in very bad condition. In a corner near the stove was a cot with curtains about it for those who were liable to die. My first day, a handsome *poilu* with thick black hair and big black eyes was brought in right from the trenches. He had both legs cut off, but fortunately, he did not know it. I stayed by his bedside most of the time after he came out of the ether, but he died at ten that night.

I became especially interested the next day in a little blond man who had been wounded three times and given every kind of decoration. He died that evening. After this I was so exhausted and sad that I hardly slept, and cried most of the night. Then I caught cold in my side, and blistered it with iodine. Indeed, I was discouraged, but kept going and didn't lose an hour's work.

In *salle* 1 we gave salt injections and *piqûres* of morphine, etc., and had blood transfusions. I mixed every known kind of drink, and fetched and carried, and made bandages *de corps*, and covered rubber rings, for most of the wounded had to sit on them in bed, and every night rubbed down a dozen *poilus* with alcohol and powder.

Of course, there was a *grandpère* in our *salle*. One always called the older ones *grandpère* or *mon vieux*. Our *grandpère* was only thirty years old, though he had a beard and looked almost any age. He was nicknamed "The Tiger," and was certainly a rough customer. His arm and leg on one side were both badly wounded, and he had a hole in his forehead besides. A Carrel tube issued from his bandaged head, and I was obliged to squirt Dakin solution into it every two hours. He called the tube his telephone and used to tell me what he heard through it; we couldn't make out exactly whether he was a little out of his mind or very original and amusing. He insisted upon calling me Anna—I don't know why—talked a great deal about his cook-stove, and said he ate rats in the trenches. The soldiers in the adjoining beds seemed to enjoy his remarks. He was given the *Croix de Guerre* one day in the hospital, and it was touching to see how pleased he was.

We did not know the names of the patients unless we looked at the tags at the foot of the beds, and called them by their numbers. Most of them were uncomplaining and wonderful, but No. 8, who was shot in the chest, groaned and complained regularly every night in the hope of getting morphine. No. 9, who had had a leg cut off, said his wife and two children had been taken by the Germans and his house

51

destroyed. No. 10 was a nice little man, put in the corner by the stove because the doctors said he could not possibly live. But he had such a brave spirit and was so determined not to die that, to the astonishment of every one, when I left the hospital he seemed to be actually gaining.

After a time, I was transferred from this *salle* to another, where we had fifty patients; these were well on the road to recovery; some were sitting up, others hobbling round, and they were allowed to smoke. My work here was changed somewhat: I took all the temperatures and marked them on the chart, as well as all the pulses, both morning and night. When the *chariot* was wheeled in for the dressings I waited on the doctors, unless they brought their French nurses with them, and occasionally did some bandaging; and if there was nothing else to do, I scrubbed the patients.

The night nurses had the most unpleasant duty, going the rounds, as they did, in the dark, draughty corridors from *salle* to *salle*, among the dead and dying men. One nurse took a shift from eight o'clock until one, another went on from one till six in the morning. This was for the entire surgical ward of several hundred patients. There were orderlies who were supposed to be on duty, but they generally went to sleep. French hospitals do not, as a rule, have a woman nurse on duty at night.

One finds all kinds and types among the French as well as among the American nurses. The motto of the army war workers might well be. Be prepared to look out for yourself in every way—nobody else has time to bother about you! I might add, or hardly to be pleasant. If one's feelings are easily hurt, one had better not go overseas.

Our *médecin-chef* was Dr. Lardenoir. I was told the French doctors operated better than others, but the French organisation of hospitals was not good. Of course, as we belonged to an *auto-chir,* which moved with the army, not like a base hospital, our arrangements were very primitive, both for patients and workers. For instance, all the water we used had to be pumped up, and it was heated in buckets on stoves in the *salle*.

An occasional shell reminded us that Cugny was very near the lines. Just before I came, the town and *château* were partly destroyed, and an *obus* struck within a few feet of our barrack. Several weeks later thirty people were killed in the village and most of the houses levelled to the ground. Not far from us was the grave of McConnell, the well-known American flyer. McConnell was buried where he fell, and part of his machine was left on the grave. The brick monument that has

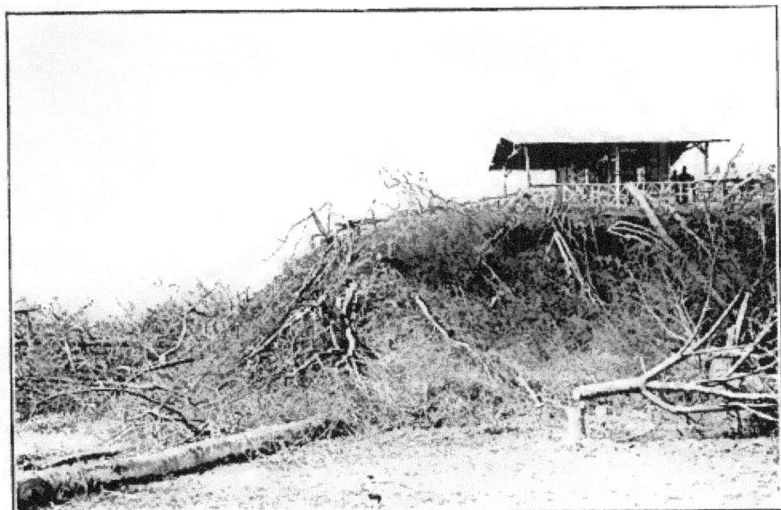

PRINCE EITEL FRIEDRICH'S OBSERVATION POST IN THE
BOIS L'ABBÉ

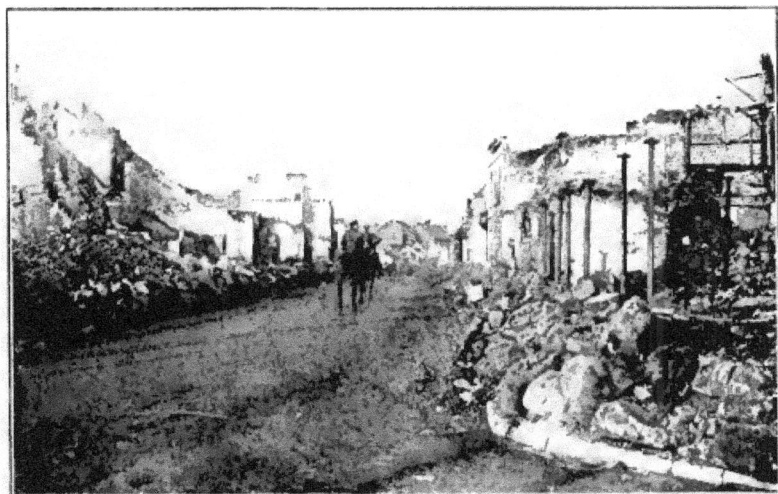

FLAVY-LE-MARTEL

been erected is decorated with flags, flowers, and his hat and gun, and the *poilus* salute as they pass by.

When the Germans overran this whole region in 1914, they erected a chalet on the top of a huge mound that rises with almost perpendicular sides above the plain not far from Cugny.

Here Prince Eitel Friedrich, the *Kaiser's* second son, used to come with his officers to drink beer and exult over his conquests. As he could survey the country for countless miles, it was well named his observation post. Elinor Glynn has thus described it:—

> It has to be approached by a path from the road now bordered by hacked-down cherry trees.

You climb to it by a steep, serpentine path with steps here and there, and a wooden balustrade in "rustic" style.

> The summit once reached, you realise immediately that you are upon a spot where Germans have imprinted their mark. A chalet stands there erected in real Teutonic taste, over the door of which is written "*Hubertushaus*," and making a circle round it are low tables with benches by them, and a quantity of those seats carved and painted to look like toadstools, which one used to see at every German health resort, and especially at Carlsbad. There is an air of theatrical unreality about the whole thing—a false note and discordant with nature.

Flavy-le-Martel was a little town a few miles nearer the trenches, to which I walked one day. Not a house was standing in the whole village. A small guard of soldiers and some American ambulance men were the only human beings quartered in the tumbling buildings.

Another day I drove from Cugny to Ham. The thirteenth-century castle here had had a huge *donjon* one hundred and ten feet high and just as wide, with enormously thick walls, which had long been used as a prison for political offenders. This is where Louis Napoleon was confined for six years after he failed at Boulogne in 1840. Nothing now remains but a great heap of stones. As I had a moment, I entered an old church, interesting because partly Romanesque, and made beautiful by the sunset light that filtered through the stained-glass windows.

The town was filled with Tommies, and the roads were gay with blue coats marching away and khaki coats marching in. The ostrich *camions* were on the move, and the different signs painted on the lorries were always amusing.

From our barrack the rattle of traffic was heard on the roads as night approached, and by the sunset light the faded blue coats of the French could be seen as they trudged along, higgledy-piggledy with their wagons and cook-stoves and their stocky, shaggy horses. The Tommies seemed bigger; they looked smarter; their uniforms were of good material and fitted well. The bagpipes played gayly as they marched down the road. It makes me very sad to think that in the spring the British here were driven back, but nothing, I believe, could have stood against the masses of Germans that rushed in at this point.

Speaking of Tommies, I had two of the nicest ones in my *salle*. They were so pleased when I gave them some of my own tea. That was not on the hospital menu, for the French preferred chocolate. One, a mere boy with blond hair, had a lady tattooed on his arm and the word "Daisy," which he laughingly insisted was his sister's name.

Mrs. Daly kindly took a few of us to dine with some French officers in a village nearby. What a wonderful dinner we had! Imagine! We had food fit for kings, in a cellar with a piano; we even had roses on the table. The *commandant* composed the most delightful poem, and we sang songs between courses. After it was over, we motored back in the darkness through the snow.

The British were about to take over this sector, and the hospital with it, so our nurses were allowed to go *en repos* for a while. Before we left a great many *blessés* were sent away to the interior. What a time we had getting them dressed! A miscellaneous collection of cleaned and mended uniforms was brought in, with an odd lot of shoes and stockings. The men passed the articles round, exchanging with each other till they finally found things that fitted. Then little presents were given them by the nurses and cheery goodbyes were said. We left them on their stretchers in the train, which was utterly dark as it pulled out into the night from the hospital platform.

Soon after this came a startling telegram. It not only startled me, but everybody else. It was from the King and Queen of Belgium, inviting me to go to Calais, where a motor would meet me and take me to the Belgian headquarters. I did not even know where the Belgian headquarters were, but was of course eager to go. That very day my husband had cabled that he hoped I might have a chance to work for the Belgians, since we had lived in Brussels before the war.

As we were going on *permission* anyway in a few days, the directress made no objection to my leaving. When she showed the telegram to the *médecin-chef*, he asked, "Who in the world is Mrs. A.? I do not know any one of that name." "She is of our *équipe*,'" the directress replied. They all seemed quite excited about it.

I had to go over to Noyon to get my *carnet rouge*—my red pass-book—signed, and the *médecin-chef* took me there in a *camion* hermetically sealed and crowded with doctors. As a properly trained nurse should, I kept respectfully silent—they perhaps thought I was French. The doctors got talking about the American troops and one said, "I don't believe the Americans know what they are up against, for they have not had much fighting. We fear they will soon be mashed into jam." On arriving, the *médecin-chef* and I walked through some quaint streets to the market-place, where the Hôtel de Ville and a church were really quite fine, and saw the *docteur général*, a pleasant old gentleman. By this time, it was dark, but we went on to the office of a captain, who signed and stamped my pass for me.

So, I went back to Cugny to get ready for my trip, which was likely to be an adventurous one. There was no telling what might happen, but I knew that at least I should soon be on my way to see the king and queen!

GRAND QUARTIER CENTRAL   G. Q. G. Belges à 22 h.50

BELGES

N° 116. 22 heure 50.

SERVICE DU ROI.

Comte de HEAY Chef du Cabinet du Roi
des Belges.

À Madame Larz ANDERSON Hopital Autochir N° 7
à CUGNY.

Leurs Majestés me chargent de vous demander s'il
vous serait possible venir les voir Vendredi ou
Samedi prochain au GRAND QUARTIER GENERAL BELGE.

Veuillez Télégraphier si pourrez arriver par
Chemin de Fer CALAIS, ou si désirez que Auto
soit envoyée à votre rencontre dans une autre
localité..

À CUGNY le 17 Janvier 1918 à 7 Heures.

THE KING'S TELEGRAM

CHAPTER 5

The Queen's Package

The night before I was to start for Calais, I took a bath, to celebrate my approaching visit to royalty, and packed my little bag, and was ready to leave at five the next morning. What happened to Germaine is still a mystery; not only did she fail to call me, but she had taken off my only pair of boots to be cleaned, and had not brought them back. However, in the pitchy blackness I reached the next barrack, awakened her and rescued my boots, snatched a piece of bread, and got a little coffee from the night nurse. Then I started off in the motor, with the two British girls, over the road lighted only by the flashing guns from Saint Quentin in the distance.

When we reached the station of Ham I paddled through the mud and got my ticket. The train left just as the sun came up in a rose-pink sky behind the skeleton of what was once a great house, outlining it black against the heavens. The huge windows of the *façade* were without glass, like large, sightless eyes. As the train went westward through the invaded section, in which only ruined towns and tottering houses were to be seen, we passed old, overgrown trenches and heaps of tangled, rusty barbed wire. (See Appendix.) On through Nesle and other towns where reconstruction work was being done, which has all been wasted, for, as everybody knows, the Boches made their terrible spring drive through Cugny and Ham, pushing back the Allied troops almost to Amiens.

As we approached that beautiful cathedral town, the country, with its canals and vegetable gardens, looked more like Holland than France. All the stations along the way were bristling with Tommies and their nice-looking officers. I found Amiens no longer a French town, but absolutely British. Not just English, but British, for there were Australians with their hats turned up on the side, and New Zealanders with hats more like our "Sammies'." Then there were East Indians in turbans and big workmen from northern China, too, with fur-lined ear-tabs on their caps. Only an occasional smart-looking French officer was left, with his bright blue uniform, fur collar, and gold braid.

The stop at Amiens was only long enough for me to get some chocolate and an omelette at a near-by restaurant and mail some postcards—which, however, never reached home—before I had to pick up my bag and board a train for the north. But, as we pulled out of the station, I caught one glimpse of the wonderful cathedral, raising its " mountainous roof" above the houses of the town, above all the hurrying soldiers brought from Far East and Far West, above all the signs of warfare—rising like a mighty rock-fortress, a symbol of the spirit of Christian civilization. I little thought that, before I returned to America, the barbarians would but just be stopped from laying sacrilegious hands on this temple, for the British during their retreat were forced to leave the way open to Amiens.

General Sandeman Carey was ordered to hold this gap until he could be relieved. He had no troops, only a few field guns—he was a general of artillery—so he had to create infantry. At two o'clock his orders came. He sent out his messengers and telephone calls, his signal-men waved their flags. A motley army came hurrying—sturdy laborers, machine-gun units, electricians, British engineers, men from the infantry training school, and finally, a company of American engineers, like all the rest, full of pluck and grit. By afternoon of the next day, this scratch force was organised and posted, and for six days they held on. It was they who kept the German Army from reaching Amiens.

On the road to the coast we passed Abbéville, an ancient fortified town, and Étaples. At last I got a glimpse of the blue sea. By the time I reached Calais, which is constantly bombed by air raids, it was quite dark. I made my way to the *Bureau* in the station to show my papers. There I spied a magnificent Belgian officer in khaki-coloured uniform, with red collar and gold braid; the man looked at least a general, but I found him to be a *commandant*. I went boldly up to him and asked if he was waiting for a Mrs. Anderson. He said he was, and soon we were whizzing along in the king's motor toward La Panne.

I shall not soon forget the courtesy of this Belgian officer, who was quite a hero. At the beginning of the war he led the cavalry at Haarlem. Then he fought with the British in the Congo, and returned, covered with medals, to be the king's *aide*.

It was an exciting trip, for when we reached Dunkirk the gates were shut because a very bad air raid was going on. It appeared I was to dine that night at seven-thirty with the king and queen, and we were even then late, so in spite of the danger the gates were opened to let the king's car through. There were at least ten searchlights playing in the heavens, and they seemed to be coming from all directions and meeting over our heads, where the Boche plane was sailing about. Rockets were bursting, too, with parachute star-lights attached. Anti-aircraft guns were banging away, and shrapnel was falling, and no doubt bombs, for all I know. I was sitting on the bottom of the motor, so that in case the glass was broken, I might not be cut, and also in order that I might gaze up into the sky and see what was going on. We passed safely through the city, however, and continued on our way to La Panne, where I was taken to the hotel to dress for dinner.

On arriving, I discovered to my horror, that my bag was not in the motor. But the maid brushed my boots, and I washed my hands, and went on as I was, in my blue nurse's uniform, to the king's house. This was a pretty villa some two miles or more from La Panne, quite by itself in a clump of trees. I was ushered into a small room to the right of the hall, where Count Van den Steen de Jehay and his wife were waiting. The count had been Minister to Luxembourg while we were living in Belgium, but as his wife had been for many years, lady-in-waiting, I had known her in Brussels.

Across the hall a door opened, and there stood the king and queen in the centre of a small sitting-room. I curtsied at the entrance. The queen put out her hand, and I curtsied again, and also to the king, as is the custom. He was in khaki with the black and red collar and the stars of the commander-in-chief of the army. She wore a simple white gown, cut V-shaped in the neck, and no jewels. They both looked extremely well, in spite of what they had been through, and both as young as I remembered them five years ago.

Her Majesty asked me in a very informal way to follow her into the dining-room. The room was small, with a round table that left rather a blue and white impression on me. My seat was on the king's left, and the countess was on my other side. I was extremely tired and very hungry, and did full credit to the simple meal of soup, fish, meat, pudding, and fruit. I had had nothing since a cup of chocolate at eleven, except the bread in my pocket.

The thing that stands out now in my mind is that the king, who looked rather solemn, surprised me by joking. He said what he remembered especially about his visit to America was the ice water that

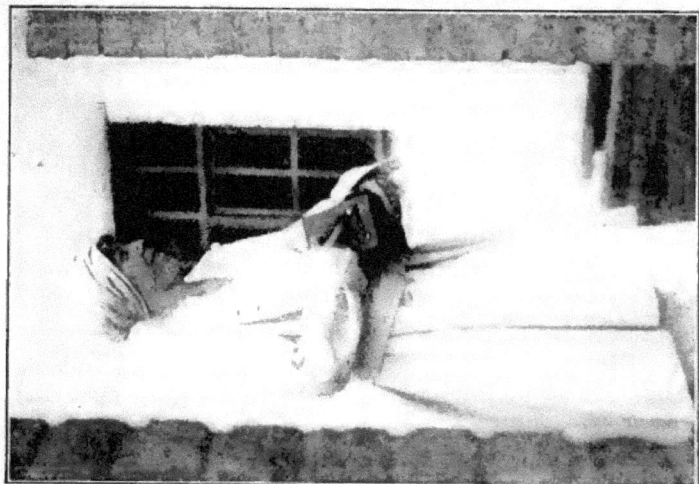

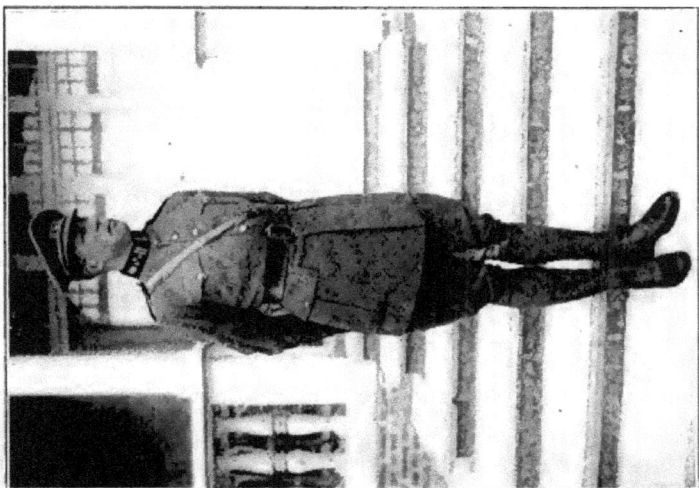

THE KING AND QUEEN OF THE BELGIANS

was given him immediately on arriving at every hotel. In regard to the war, when I asked if the Belgian Congo troops were to be sent for, he remarked that he did not approve of the different races being brought into the country, that the Chinese workmen had already made some trouble, that, curiously enough, they were marrying European women. When I spoke about the Japanese, His Majesty said they were different, as they were such good fighters.

After dinner, while the king and the count went off into another room to smoke, and the countess went to call up Lady Hadfield on the telephone,—an old friend of mine who was running the Anglo-American hospital for British officers at Wimereux,—the queen and I had quite a long talk in the little parlour, all by ourselves. She was very simple and sweet and bright, and told me a good many interesting things, speaking in English and in the very low voice which royalty seems always to use. After a while. King Albert came back and said he wanted his *aide* to take me in a motor the next day to Dr. Depage's hospital and also to see some of the destroyed villages; that his *aide* had arranged for me to visit an American woman who ran a canteen not far from the trenches, and that Lady Hadfield had telephoned she expected me at Wimereux to stay with her for a few days.

The queen asked if I would like to go into the trenches, and of course I jumped at the suggestion. The king wondered if my husband would object, and wanted to know what clothes I would wear at the front. I was obliged to tell Their Majesties I had nothing but my uniform for my bag had been left at Calais. Then it was decided that the little fur cap I had tucked in my pocket and my trench coat which made me look much like a man, would do very well. The queen said that only two other women had been in the Belgian trenches. The queen herself has been often to the front, even into the first-line trenches; she certainly is a heroine and an inspiration to her people.

The king and queen left the room at the end of the evening, after saying many pleasant things about America and sending messages to my husband. I told them how enthusiastic the Americans were over Their Majesties, and spoke of my desire to work for the Belgians, and of the chance that it might be possible to do so during my *permission* with the French. They said they hoped it could be arranged, and that perhaps I could work at Dr. Depage's hospital or at the countess's cousin's near Poperinghe. The count asked me to sign in their visitors' book. Before the war this was filled with German royalties. The King and Queen of Italy had visited them recently. Then the *commandant* came with the motor to take me back to the tiny hotel in La Panne.

As I was leaving the palace, to my surprise a little package was handed me, in which I found a nightgown of the queen's, a comb and brush, soap, and several handkerchiefs! It was thoughtful and kind of Her Majesty to do this, and I appreciated everything, especially the handkerchiefs, for I had a cold.

The little inn was filled with men playing the piano and singing. I went to sleep with rollicking soldier songs in my ears. In the morning the *commandant* came for me, and we went to Dr. Depage's hospital. An old hotel, built directly on the beach at La Panne, had been made ready by Madame Depage for her husband's use, early in the war. Then many temporary pavilions had been put up nearby, in the town. Now Ocean Hospital, as it was called, contained five hundred beds and was considered a model. The officers' quarters were in the main building; there I discovered a Count D'Ursel, whom I had known before and who had lived on the same street with us in Brussels. He had been wounded in the leg, but was almost well. He told me he was expecting his *fiancée*, and that they were to be married soon in La Panne.

After that Dr. Depage took me from one great pavilion filled with gay, chintz-covered beds to another. It all looked very clear and cheerful, and was apparently full. I noticed especially a number of gas patients, who lay coughing, with their eyes covered, for the gas affects both eyes and lungs.

In the operating-room a doctor was amputating a leg. He told us the soldier had a bad case of gangrene, and he was obliged to cut off the leg very high up. The man was, of course, under the influence of chloroform. How dreadful it seemed! Little did I think I should soon be working in that very same room myself and seeing such cases every day!

Dr. Depage showed me electric devices for heating the patients in bed, and a bed on wheels which an American doctor had made for him, and a little cutting machine for making compresses—this device certainly saves labour, and all the time I worked there I never saw any frayed edges. If there were any, they could be quickly taken out by the nurse before the surgeon used the compresses. After seeing this machine, it seems to me rather useless for women all over the United States to put so much time and labour into a thing that can be done so quickly and well by machinery. When I remarked this to an American woman in charge of surgical dressings, her answer was, "American doctors are so particular." But I certainly think there is a great deal to be said in favour of the machine.

Then I was shown a new ambulance with only one bed in it, which was on springs; Dr. Depage said the King of England had been carried in this ambulance when he fell from his horse, and had liked it so much that he had ordered a number for the British Army.

The instruments and the artificial legs that are made at this hospital interested me greatly. Dr. Depage feels that in order to keep the correct balance, the artificial leg should be the same weight and the same shape as the natural leg that has been cut off, which is quite a new idea.

We went through kitchens, laboratories, and laundry—we saw everything, in fact—and then had luncheon at Dr. Depage's villa nearby, looking out over the long white beach with green-grey water breaking along the edge. The doctor was good enough to say he would like me to remain as an *infirmière*. As that was exactly what I wanted to do, we sat down and wrote out a telegram to Mrs. Daly, and it was decided that I should wait at Lady Hadfield's for an answer.

After luncheon the *commandant* and I started off again in the motor, stopping first at the picturesque old town of Furnes, with its beautiful square fronted by the Hôtel de Ville and the old tower. Peter Titelmann the Inquisitor must often have stalked across this Grande Place, in the days when in the sacred name of religion, he was torturing and burning the devoted Flemings.

Above the quaint little brick houses rose the partly demolished church of Saint Walburge, a huge torso of a choir with neither nave nor transepts. Only a very few houses were occupied, used as wine and cake shops for the soldiers; though the town was battered, these people still remained, either because they had no place to go, or they wished to make a little money.

My escort told me that at one time in the early part of the war, King Albert had been in the Hôtel de Ville when two German officers were brought in prisoners and taken before him. The king asked one of them why it was that the Germans bombarded beautiful old towns simply to kill a few innocent women and children. The officer's answer was that His Majesty was mistaken, that the Germans never did that, but just as the words came out of his mouth, a bomb dropped in the square.

We went on in the rain past smaller villages, quite in ruins, out through the deep mud, over the flat country, by trenches and barbed wire and canals and mud huts and cement caves, past guns covered by greens and ammunition camouflaged with turf, and soldiers quartered in haystacks. How history repeats itself! This plain of Flanders, we are told:

> In the seventeenth century was so studded with earthen redoubts and serrated by long lines of field-works and ditches that the whole countryside between Ypres and Dunkirk was virtually a vast entrenched camp.

The *commandant* showed me a little church where fifty Alpine *chasseurs* had been housed for a night, but a bomb had struck it, and all had been killed. We passed small companies of Belgian soldiers marching along the road, and motor *camions*, and army kitchens drawn by horses. He explained that only a few soldiers marched together, so that if a shot fell, many would not be killed at once.

Suddenly, in turning the corner of a narrow street, along which only the walls of a few houses were standing, the motor stopped terrifically short, and there was a terrible bang. I must say that for the first time I felt myself growing white, for it seemed, as if we must be struck by a German shell. But we instantly discovered six Belgian soldiers firing a big cannon in the street. Little did they expect to see a motor in this region, and still less a woman, and they were as much surprised as we. The road which we followed after leaving the village was supposed to be hidden by high bushes, but the Boches evidently knew it was there, for the ground on either side was covered with hundreds of *obus* holes. It was shelled principally at night, when the troops moved.

We finally arrived at the River Yser, below Dixmude, the last town we left being Nieuw Cappelle. The canal and the river flow higher than the level country; behind the dikes are the trenches of wood and mud. On account of the flat, muddy country the soldiers' quarters are built up above the surface, and so are quite unlike the ordinary, deep, zigzag trenches.

Some quarters had wooden floors and beds and tables—one officer's room even had a telephone and a chair. Some of the others, however, had no floor and only straw and a blanket for furnishings. At this point there was a bend in the river and a sand bar at one side; on the other side of the river were the Boches, among some trees—we were less than half a mile away, in what they called the first-line trenches; we crept up on the bank behind a tree and I had a good view of the flat country. It appears the Germans seldom pick off a single person with a rifle in the daytime—at least, we are still alive. I hope this verse of a "rhyme from a new nursery" is true:—

> *There was a little Hun,*
> *And he had a little gun,*
> *And his bullets were all dumdum, dumdum;*
> *He shinned up a tree*
> *To snipe what he could see,*
> *But now he is in Kingdom come-come-come!"*

It was astonishing to find, so near the front lines, a tiny farmhouse, half demolished, hidden under the bank, where an old woman and a rosy-cheeked peasant girl lived, with their three cows. The *commandant* said that they had been ordered away time and time again, but they had sent letters to the king saying they wished to remain—they had no place to go, and they made a little money selling milk to the soldiers—so he had allowed them to stay.

While we were there, many shells, both German and Belgian, whizzed by over our heads. Some we could even see as they landed about two hundred yards away, and could hear the splash and see the mud fly. This was not exactly a place to linger in. On our way back, while the motor was rocking and jumping in the ruts, a glorious sunset was lighting up the whole region.

At Loo, where the big church was tottering, we came at last to a few tents and a wee portable house—of wood, but much like our portable houses of tin—where I found a woman from Boston whom I knew, seated by a stove in a pleasant sitting-room and having tea. We arrived at the right moment to congratulate her, for it appeared she had been decorated that day. She was in Belgium at the beginning of the war, first in hospital work, and then in canteen. This worker and the two British women at Pervyse are the only ones who have been allowed to remain so near the trenches as far as I know, for an order went out from the Allies that women should not be given permission to work just behind the lines.

One of her tents, used as a reading-room, contained comfortable chairs for the soldiers, the daily newspapers, Flemish and French, the weekly illustrated papers, and books, also writing-tables, where paper was supplied free of charge.

Another tent had nothing but games, such as checkers, chess and cards, and musical instruments—concertina, violin, *mandolin* and flute. When we entered this tent, all the soldiers sprang to their feet and stood at attention. The directress then asked one of them to play for us on a violin, and he did so, quite delightfully, for the Belgians are very musical. Every evening, she played the gramophone to them, much to their delight.

In still another tent, tea, coffee, cocoa and crackers were served to the men over a counter. The directress also had six annexes for the use of the artillery men, who were obliged to remain with their guns. These annexes were run quite the same, except that everything was in miniature, the library having only twenty-five books, which were changed every two weeks.

On we motored in the darkness through Dunkirk to Calais, where I found my bag, and along the sand dunes on the coast till we reached the Anglo-American hospital at Wimereux. There we found Lady Hadfield, who had a nice dinner waiting for us by a cheerful fire. I said goodbye to the *commandant*, who went back to La Panne, while I remained in this delightful, homelike place for a whole week among the British. (See Appendix.)

CHAPTER 6

The British Base

The huge city of tents reaching for many miles along the coast was like the British Empire transported to France. There were English and Canadian, Australian and New Zealand hospitals, rest camps, and convalescent camps, and horse camps, to say nothing of the hospitals for the officers and the clubhouses, the experimental wards for flying men, and the innumerable plants needed for the upkeep of them all. Everything British is on such a tremendous scale that you are over-whelmed by the mere size of it. There is hardly a hospital with less than two thousand beds. I asked Colonel B. what points should be emphasised in organising a hospital; to which he replied that it was more economical to have it on a large scale—not under one thousand beds, and two thousand or more preferably. (See Appendix.)

Out of the twenty-two base hospitals, organised and equipped by the American Red Cross, five were back of the British lines, when I was there, and were among the first to be sent from this country fol-lowing the entry of the United States into war. The personnel of a five hundred-bed hospital unit consists of a commanding officer from the Army Medical Corps; a quartermaster, twenty-two doctors, two den-tists, sixty-five nurses, one hundred and fifty-three men of the enlisted Reserve Corps of the Medical Department of the Army; six civilian employees, including a registrar, a dietitian, laboratory technicians and stenographers; and a chaplain.

The British organisation is in general respects like the French, in that they have dressing-stations and army doctors just behind the lines. Their ambulance posts are farther back. The evacuation hospitals are about eight miles from the trenches, and their base miles away. The hospital ships carry some of the wounded to Blighty. I saw a train unloading near the docks and the cripples being carried on stretchers

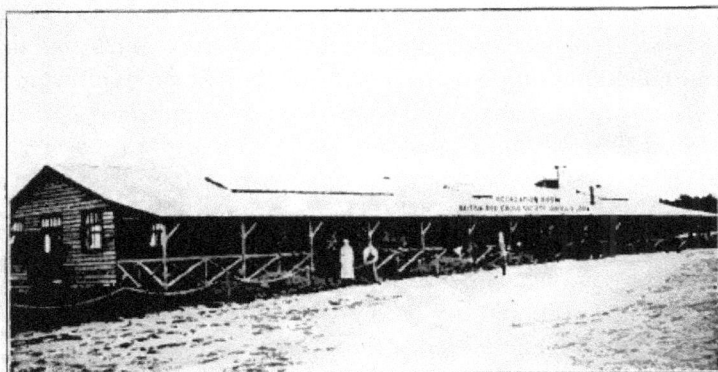

THE BRITISH RED CROSS HUT AT A CONVALESCENT DEPOT

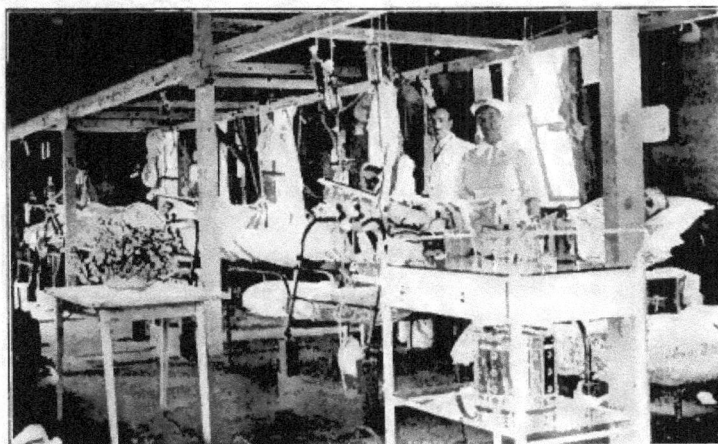

IN A BRITISH BASE HOSPITAL

to the camouflaged ship. This train was remarkably well fitted up, with its bunks, private rooms, office, kitchen and operating-room, nurses and doctors.

Unlike the French, the English have kept their best surgeons at the bases, but lately they are changing their point of view and are doing what the French have done since the beginning of the war, that is, they are putting their best ones at the evacuation hospitals. Outside, their barracks, or huts, as they call them, look very much like those of the French. But inside there are differences. The pretty flowing veil of the *infirmière* is replaced by a cap. One no longer hears, "*Bonjour, mademoiselle!*" or "*Bonjour, grandpère,*" or "*Mon vieux, tu vas bien*"; now it is, "The top of the morning to you, Sister," or "How are you feeling. Daddy?" or "Goodnight, Jock." There are among the British many V.A.D.'s,—nurses' aids,—who are proving a great success in spite of their shorter training. I am glad to hear we are now beginning to send American aids over, for they are needed. (*Vide The V.A.Ds* by Maud Mortimer, Olive Dent & Thekla Bowser; Leonaur 2014.)

The French and Belgians are obliged to employ a great many nuns and *infirmières* without diplomas because few, if any, diplomaed nurses are to be had among them. I know Dr. Depage was the first to introduce the system of training nurses in Brussels a few years before the war, and there was much controversy over it. Nuns had always done the work, and at that time many people considered them quite sufficient. British and American nurses are not allowed as near the front lines as the French and Belgian women, except on British hospital trains going to the front, which I should think one of the most interesting posts of all, and at the advanced operating centres during a battle.

The officers' hospital at Wimereux, where I stayed with Lady Hadfield, is a perfect little place, pretty and clean and homelike, with a large ward downstairs and private rooms above. Lady Hadfield had a bedroom and sitting-room of her own, and I was installed in her guest-room which seemed like heaven after my experience in the barracks at Cugny. The night I arrived, there were many officers in the entrance hall, lying silently on stretchers covered with blankets, while an orderly went quietly from one to another, writing down their names and the nature of their wounds.

Lady Hadfield, who is an American, is an attractive woman and an excellent executive. She started this institution at the beginning of the war, and has certainly earned the decorations which have been given her for her long, steady work. Whether indoors or out, she can always be recognised, for she never wears anything but white. At first her house was for Tommies, but it has lately been turned over to officers, and is called Anglo-American because it is open to Americans as well. It is supported by her own private means, but the sisters are supplied by the British Red Cross.

Wimereux, like Étretat and La Panne, was once a lovely French seaside resort with hotels, restaurants, and pretty villas where the rich amused themselves. Now it is almost like a part of British territory, and one scarcely hears French spoken anywhere. The streets are filled with lively Tommies and Waacs.

These Waacs, of whom there are thousands, are sometimes called Brownies and sometimes Chocolate Drops, and are the paid women workers of the war. They are principally employed in offices of various kinds and in all the industries where they can take the place of men. For instance, I saw many of them working as printers. One of the girls told me they had been selected from bookbinding houses in London and that they were paid seven dollars a week and given good food. Most of them lived in huts, which had curved corners to save lumber, and did not have much light or look very comfortable. Counting the Waacs as well as the nursing sisters, there were about ten thousand English women in France at that time. As a whole they are a fine set of workers. (See Appendix.) Indeed, the women of England in general stand out splendidly in this war. The French, curiously enough, thought that the British idea in importing so many of them was to prevent the Tommies from marrying foreigners and to keep the race Anglo-Saxon.

We motored over one day to Le Touquet, where we went to the casino, which is now a perfect hospital for officers, run by the Duchess of Westminster. In the old days, it was a gay gambling house, but now one sees quite a different scene. What a wonderful place to get well in, among the sweet-smelling pines, with the salt breeze blowing in from the sea!

Passing through some scrubby woods, we got a view of a number of ugly summer houses perched upon the dunes. There are lovely walks, however, through pine forests, and in days before the war there were little casinos here and there, where tea and chocolate could be taken. We stopped to watch the superb sunset over the water and the incoming tide as it devoured the wide, hard beach.

Very near Wimereux is the old French port of Boulogne, with its ancient church and heavy walls. Of late it had completely changed its

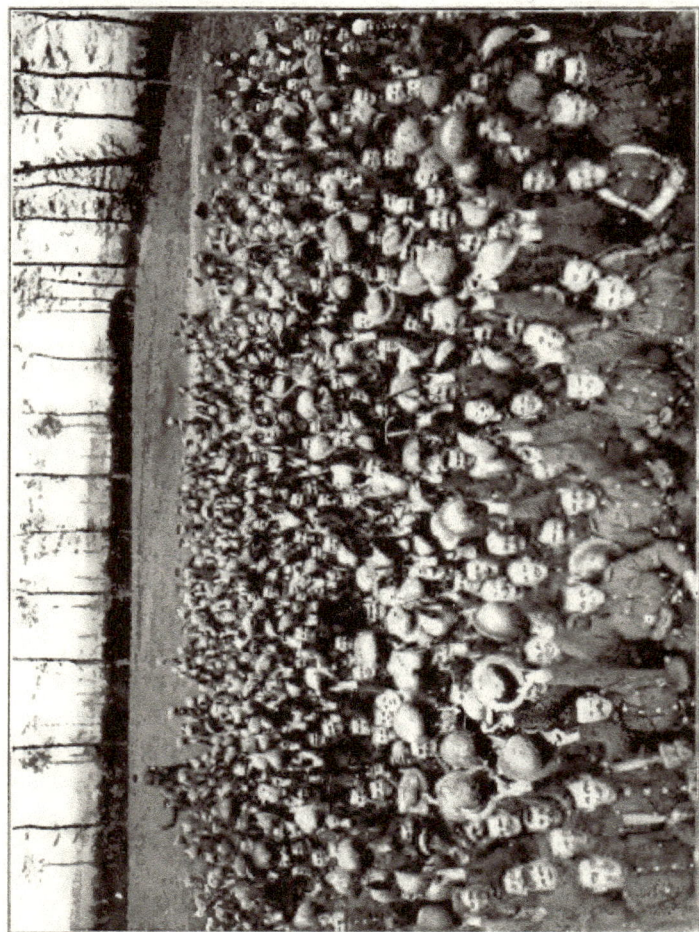

A BATTALION OF THE MIDDLESEX REGIMENT (DIE HARDS)

life as well as its language. The shop windows now looked sporty to tempt the Tommies; the old French town no longer slept but almost danced with activity. The hotels and houses here were so crowded that the officers' clubhouse—built of corrugated iron and painted red—was much appreciated. It was for those on the move, and was fitted with cubicles with pretty bed covers and curtains. The dining-room and tables were gay with flowers, and there were nice-looking waitresses. The sitting-room seemed comfortable and homelike. The charge was only seven *francs* fifty per day.

Number 13, an American Red Cross hospital, had some of our best doctors on its staff, Dr. Harvey Gushing, for instance, so celebrated for operating on heads. It was originally a large casino near the mouth of the river. It had about eight hundred beds, was old and rather dark, but most of the wounded were put on the lower floor, and for that reason it was convenient for shipping convalescents to England.

Sir Almeroth Wright, the noted bacteriologist, we found here experimenting in his laboratory to determine the first moment when it is best to close a wound. If a wound could be sewed up more quickly than is done today and still heal, it would be a great saving of work and expense. We found Sir Almeroth very humorous and delightful.

In the ward for the aviators at another institution were a captured German machine and a new contrivance to determine the condition of an aviator's heart. Many of them develop weak hearts, and nervous disorders, and are seldom good fliers afterwards. Up to this time the English had never examined their bird-men so thoroughly.

Two great bakeries at Boulogne fed over half a million soldiers. Men had been employed here, but they were being replaced by women. The flour was mixed and worked by hand in great tubs, then shoved by ladles into trays, and from these into huge ovens; when taken out the loaves were stacked and counted, and finally packed in sacks, forty in a sack. The kneading of the bread was hard work, and putting it in and taking it out of the furnace was a hot, disagreeable task, but much of it was to be done in the future by machinery. Twelve hundred persons were employed in one of these bakeries, and seven were killed a short time ago, when it was struck by a bomb.

One fat, round loaf was enough for two soldiers' rations for a day. The shape of the loaves and the quality of the bread was quite different from that of the French. I tasted it and found it very good. The general who was with us presented me with a loaf; the bread used in the army was whiter and better than workers could get at the base.

The general also took me into the huge refrigerating plant, where we saw great pieces of meat from Argentina, done up in sacking. Two of these plants stored enough for half a million men. It was put in food trains or lorries with bread, tea, cereals and jam, and sent to the front, where all was eaten by the soldiers in the trenches three days later. This showed the fine organisation of the British behind the lines, which was not equalled by any other country.

At Wimereux there are historical associations on every hand. Nearby on a high hill is the *Colonne de la Grande Armée*, to which we motored. On this site Napoleon assembled an army to invade England in 1804. But he waited in vain for the French fleets, for Britain's navy was then, as always, her protection, and Nelson's victory at Trafalgar put an end to all thoughts of invasion. I climbed to the top of the column, which commanded a wide view over the enormous camps and across the stormy Channel, and listened to the cannon on the front.

Only a few miles away was Guînes, to which came long ago the two great rivals, Henry VIII of England and Francis I of France, each hoping to outshine the other by his gorgeous display on the Field of the Cloth of Gold. I tried to imagine the scene:—

Guînes at that time still belonged to England, and just outside its castle was erected the enormous palace of wood and glass, hung with silks and velvets and Arras tapestries, where Henry was to receive the French Court. Near the adjoining town of Ardres were the three hundred tents of the French nobles, covered with cloth of gold and of silver, in the centre of which stood the huge gilded tent of their king. Their queens and all the greatest lords of their realms attended the monarchs to the place of meeting.

The two gorgeous camps were on opposite slopes, and between them in the valley was a little stream which formed the dividing line. Down to this rode the two kings—Henry, robust and rosy-cheeked, in cloth of silver gleaming with jewels, the tall, handsome Francis magnificent in cloth of gold. They spurred their steeds to a gallop as they drew near each other, then reined up suddenly side by side, saluted, embraced, dismounted from their horses, and arm in arm walked to a great golden pavilion, where Cardinal Wolsey and Admiral Bonnivet were waiting to do them homage. A treaty was signed here, and for three weeks games and tournaments were celebrated in lists of unheard-of splendour.

Impressive in a different way was the vast expanse of British tents, stretching for miles along the shore, which met my eyes as I turned

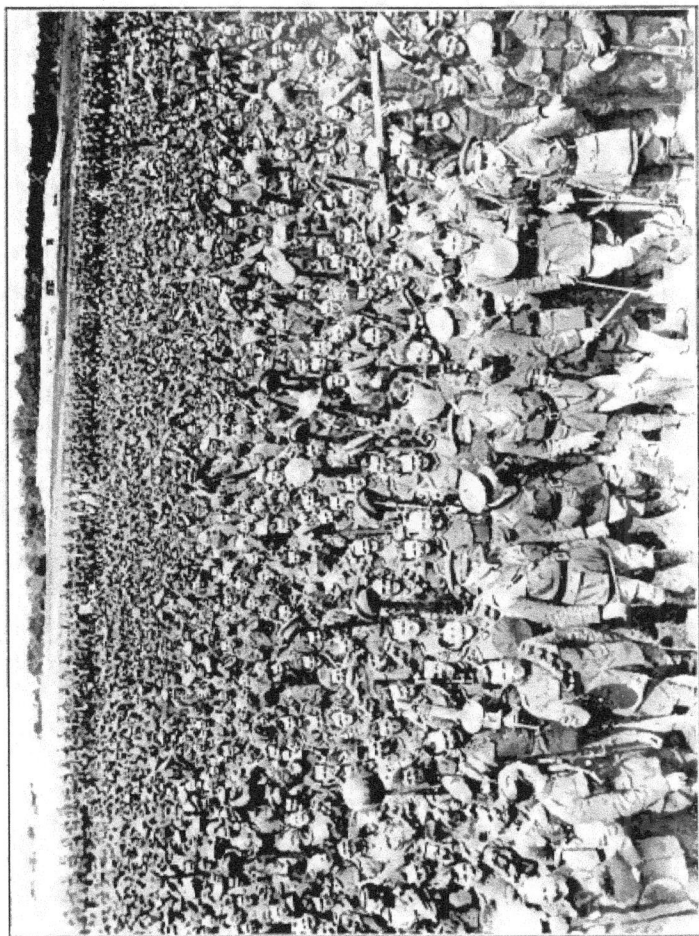

A BRITISH TRAINING SCHOOL ON THE WESTERN FRONT

my gaze toward the coast. On the top of the cliff not far away was the huge convalescent camp, which had its clubs and recreation halls and night lunchrooms. Every kind of trade was carried on there. Old shoes and clothes were mended; there were baths and laundry and disinfecting plant, all the work done by soldiers who knew the trade before. They were only kept, as a rule, for three months and then sent back to the trenches. The dispensary and kitchens were economically run; for instance, the fat was all saved and much of it sent back to England. A marvellous institution it was, of great credit to Colonel Campbell.

We motored past gas stations, where they tested different sorts of gas and where soldiers were shown how to protect themselves with masks. And we had a look at the camp full of horses, sick or wounded but worth trying to save. As a Tommy expressed it, "They are taken care of as well as babies."

Everything is done in a lavish way among the British for their soldiers and workers, who certainly deserve it. The French are more economical, as they have always been, and as perhaps they are obliged to be.

In talking with a colonel who had charge of seven German prison camps I was told that if a prisoner escaped and was caught, he was given fourteen days in the guardhouse. The prisoners were well fed, so they worked well, he said, and made little trouble, but had to be closely guarded because they tried to escape. In these prison enclosures at the base, surrounded as usual by a barbed wire, each man slept alone in order to prevent them from communicating with one another. They were employed principally in working on the roads. Those I saw looked in good physical condition, and their clothes were clean and mended.

If they refused to work, they were shipped by the French officers into the interior with the order that they should be given nothing but bread and water until they went about their tasks. Others I saw in France seemed happy and polite, and did their work well. They were so far from the lines that it would have been difficult for them to escape, but they told me they were well fed and well treated, and they looked as if they were. The German wounded in the hospitals, both in France and Belgium, had the same care as the other patients, the only difference being that they had their beds together at one side and were not mixed with their enemies.

One afternoon I strolled out on the beach and watched the fisher folk; the women with full short skirts were wading barefooted among the rocks, looking for shellfish. The fishing trade had been badly damaged, although a few boats painted grey could be seen off the shore. The high brown cliffs rose on either side of the beach, and a mediaeval tower stood out of the blue sea, while the sun setting behind it turned the misty sky to the colour of a pink and mauve hydrangea.

My leave was up, and no answer had come to my telegram to Mrs. Daly—indeed, having discovered that telegrams appeared to be even more uncertain than letters and often longer in coming, I decided to start for Paris and find out what was expected of me.

The last night at Wimereux was an exciting one. After a delightful little dinner, it was suggested that since it was such a superb moonlight evening we should go out on the beach. All accordingly wandered down toward the sea and had just reached the *plage* when suddenly searchlights began to play in the heavens, and anti-aircraft guns banged and shrapnel fell about us. A raid was on! We hurried under the eaves of a house and then gradually made our way home to the hospital, dodging in the vestibules on the way. As far as I know, only one bomb was dropped, and that was in Boulogne and did not kill anyone. The next morning, I was off on the train for Paris.

CHAPTER 7

Town and Trench

No sooner had I reached Paris than the telegram was forwarded from Mrs. Daly, saying that I might remain in Belgium Libre and work at Dr. Depage's hospital during my *permission*! Of course, the first thing to do was to get back there as soon as possible, but this was not so easily done, as the question of passes is always complicated. Hurrying to the Belgian Legation, I tried to get into communication with Dr. Depage and the *inspecteur général*, Dr. Mélis, but there were so many delays that it began to look as if all my *permission* would be used up in getting the pass for La Panne.

Not wishing to remain idle during my leave, I ran from pillar to post, trying to find something to do, feeling like a desperate servant looking for a situation. The trouble was, I preferred to work at the front, and apparently to offer one's services there for a few weeks was like asking for a diamond necklace.

Once I had an offer to go to a hospital for *poilus* at Evereux, run by an American. A friend of mine was there, and the directress telegraphed me to come. I was all packed up to go when another wire arrived, saying that a new rule would not permit aids to serve for so short a time.

Determined to go somewhere, I didn't much care where, I was very much pleased when a chance came to start a diet kitchen very near the trenches. But just at that point, who should turn up but Dr. Depage himself!

"If I can arrange matters, would you like to go back to La Panne with me in the motor?" he asked.

As this was what I wanted above everything else, and as he was able to "arrange matters" with astonishing ease, it was no time at all before my bags were piled into his car and we were off for Ocean Hospital.

My few days in Paris had not been wasted, by any means. Being a forehanded person, I took advantage of the leisure moment to pack my steamer trunk for America with my few souvenirs and some things which would not be needed. My clothes were in a frightful state, and I was obliged to send for Gabrielle, a little French maid, to come in and clean and mend them, while I did some necessary shopping. Not very much, however, as one is not allowed to take home more than one brings over. (I was warned, by the way, not to take other people's parcels or letters.)

Some long-delayed letters and marvellous packages arrived from home—just the things I needed and found so hard to get—candy and cigarettes, stockings, sweaters and boots. Among these things were some of my Christmas presents, which I received in March.

Then, since I was doing no work, it seemed a good moment to arrange the papers for my return home. My passport read for France only, but my plan was to go back by way of England when the time came. Never did I work harder in any hospital or canteen than in getting that change made. The Americans are just as slow and just as involved in red tape as the French, if not more so.

My first attempt was at the American Embassy. They sent me to the Consulate. At the Consulate they told me to go back to the embassy. The doorkeeper there sent me on to the Navy Department. The Navy Department ordered me to the army. There I found a friend, and thought my troubles were over. But he directed me to the Red Cross. Here I was given a document permitting me to return to America by way of England. The consul's clerk took the paper to stamp it with the seal of official approval and—promptly lost it. (The consulate was being moved at the time.)

At this point the ambassador took pity on me and said he would allow the embassy to stamp my passport. But at the consulate the clerk said they did not stamp papers until three days before Americans left France, and kindly added that there were only three more places to go to, all just before sailing. What was the use of being angry? I got back to my room and sank into a chair exhausted, and had a good laugh over it all.

But the climax came on reaching Belgium Libre, where the police not only asked the usual questions regarding my age, nationality, etc., but demanded a print of my thumb! By this time I realised that I had not lived up to what was expected of me. I should at least have stolen state papers or killed my grandmother's cousin.

That trip to La Panne with Dr. Depage was one to remember. Straight north from Paris we motored, through Chantilly, with its race-track and its *château* that used to belong to a Bourbon, where there were green, level gardens and fountains and long *vistas* of clipped trees, to Amiens, that ancient, much-desired city with its thirteenth-century cathedral rising still unharmed in its midst. William Morris writes:

> It rises up from the ground, grey from the paving of the street, the cavernous portals of the west front opening wide and mar-vellous with the shadows of the carving you can only guess at; and above stand the kings, and above that you would see the twined mystery of the great flamboyant rose window with its thousand openings, and the shadows of the flower work carved round it; then the grey towers and gable; . . . and behind them all, rising high into the quivering air, the tall spire over the crossing.

Over cobble-stoned streets between high walls, or through strange roads lined with trees, the doctor directed the chauffeur, now this way, now that. Everywhere I found their roads much better than ours here at home, in spite of the heavy traffic of the *camions*. Climate and politics make a bad combination for our American road builders to meet.

By the roadside were French and English soldiers, Chinese work-men, and Boche prisoners. It was said that, not long ago, the British lighted up a prison camp in these parts at night, and German aviators, mistaking it for an English camp, bombed it. As the Chinese quarters were close by, several Chinamen were killed too, and the survivors were so angry with the Germans for bombing them that they tried to get into the prison camp and kill those that were there.

Through part of the district invaded in 1914 and again last spring, we crossed the line into Belgium Libre at Leysèle. About sunset we got a puncture, and while the chauffeur mended it we sat down by the roadside and ate our few meagre sandwiches. As night came on and we neared the front, we saw a great fire in the distance, and the flash-ing of guns and searchlights, and heard the roaring of cannon.

For some distance we ran parallel with the trenches, at one point only about four miles back, through bombarded towns, past endless lines of motor lorries—I never saw so many in my life. At this time the British were holding this part of the line, and soldiers were stationed at crossroads in towns. But they never stopped us, because painted on our motor were the magic letters, S.M.B.—*Service Militaire Beige*. It was eleven o'clock when at last we reached La Panne and had a quiet little supper beside the fire in Dr. Depage's villa by the sea.

It was decided that I should live in the house next door to Dr. Depage's and take my meals at his table. He kept open house, and had all kinds of people there, including the queen, generals, actresses, and private soldiers. He was especially nice to Americans, and a number of American doctors came to watch his methods. They all said this was a model hospital.

The conversation at table was certainly varied. Interesting, too, what I could catch of it, for it was in all kinds of French, and very rapidly spoken. Every sort of thing was discussed—food, catgut, rubber gloves, the theatre, the war, the general's leg, or the latest operation.

Two other doctors lived in the same house with Dr. Depage—one for lung and stomach wounds, the other for fractures. The wife of the physician who had charge of the head wounds ran the uniform department for the nurses; as this couple had no children of their own, they had adopted three Belgian orphans; the girl and one boy had gone to school, but the third child, a dear little curly-headed fellow about eight, they had living with them.

The morning after my arrival, I donned my new uniform and went to work at Ocean Hospital. The costume of the Belgian nurses was quite the best-looking I had seen—blue cotton dress, white apron and veil, and starched white cuffs, collar and belt.

The hospital took in all cases that came up in this section, civil as well as military. Among the patients were a number of women and children who had been bombed. The system on which it was run, dominated by the strong personality of our *médecin-chef*, was remarkable in its efficiency.

The doctor, who was head and colonel of the Belgian Red Cross, was often called the Emperor of La Panne. He really did rule the place in a way, too. A big man in every sense of the word, he sometimes rode roughshod over people who got in his way, but the whole life of La Panne, social as well as hospital, was kept going through his efforts.

Our matron was English, and there were about twenty American nurses of all types—or perhaps I should call them aids, as most of them were not diplomaed. Several had come over with Dr. Moody's unit, and when he became ill Dr. Depage took them on, and a quantity of splendid hospital material also. There were about a score of English sisters, too, at first, but they were withdrawn some time before I left because the British, it was said, considered the hospital too near the front and feared that when the spring drive commenced it would become too dangerous. (A short time before I got there a bomb had hit the hospital and killed half a dozen people.)

The other nurses were Belgians. Like the Americans, they were given food, uniforms, rooms, and laundry free, but while our women gave their services, they received a small pay in addition to their expenses.

Connected with the hospital was a large hall where either a lecture or a concert was given nearly every night, and three dramatic performances every fortnight, so that all who wished to go should have a chance. The entire hospital staff was invited to attend these entertainments, as well as soldiers billeted at La Panne, and of course the *blessés*. There were two long rows of beds across the front of the hall for those too ill to sit up.

The conductor of the Monnaie, the opera house at Brussels, was stationed at La Panne, and he discovered a number of musicians among the soldiers, so that we had excellent performances. Some of the best plays were given—*Mlle, de Beulemans*, for instance, which had such a success in Paris and Brussels.

The Belgians whom I met and worked with here were not the type of the old aristocracy whom I knew in Brussels, and who were so very Roman Catholic in the days before the war. The doctors were not particularly religious, and showed a tendency toward very liberal democracy.

Among the visitors in La Panne was an American who came, toward the end of March, to distribute Christmas boxes which had not even then arrived! A box took a month to reach me from Paris, though one could make the trip in a motor in seven hours. Boulogne is only two hours away, and yet it took another box two months to reach a friend of mine in La Panne. So, it was no wonder the Christmas presents were three months late in coming over from England, where they had been purchased.

This man told me that the boxes weighed four pounds apiece, and contained chocolate, baked beans, Quaker Oats, and jam. Now the Belgian soldiers were well fed by their government, and I wished the cripples in the hospital might have been given presents instead, for many of them had no houses and no money, and no friends to send them things.

I did enjoy the view from my little room, which was two flights up and looked out over the endless yellow beach with the white breakers, and the tides rushing in and out. When the tide was out the *plage* made

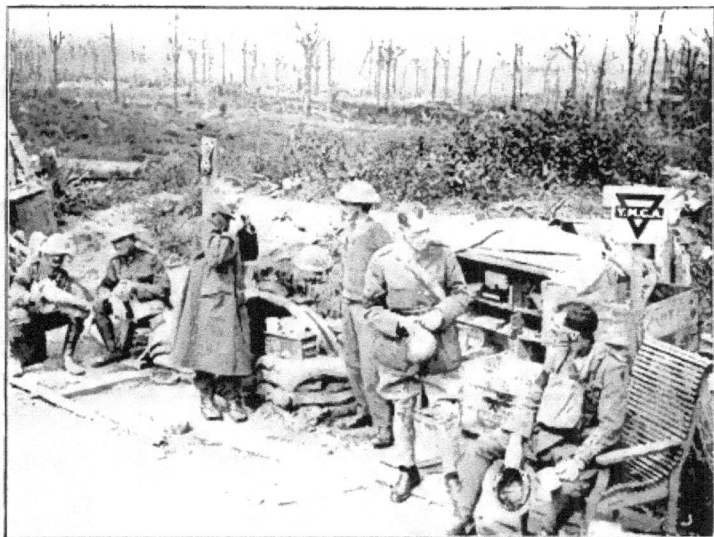

AN ADVANCED Y.M.C.A. "HUT" WHICH IS WELL UNDER
SHELL-FIRE

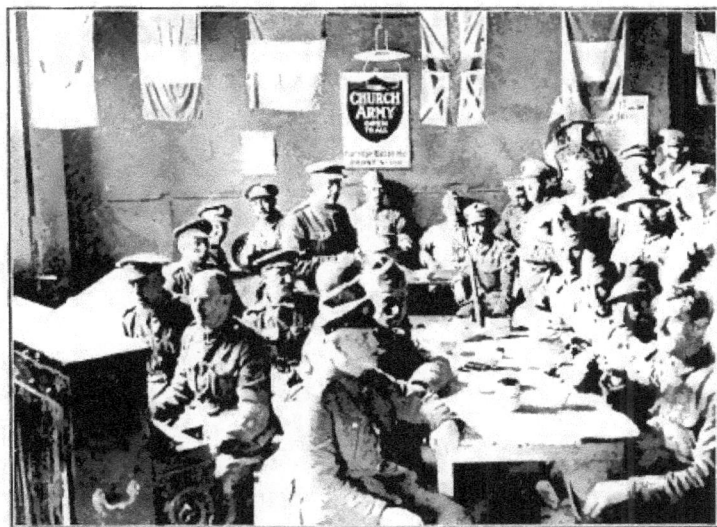

BRITISH AND FRENCH SOLDIERS HAVING A "SING-SONG"
AT A CHURCH ARMY DEPOT

a splendid parade ground, and the Belgian soldiers often drilled there.

The cavalry was always particularly stirring. The horses were brown and with the men in khaki grouped closely together, you could hardly see them against the sand were it not for the flashing of their sabres when they made a charge. Khaki is a very good colour for fighting there in winter, among the dunes and the brown mud and the dark, leafless bushes that form a camouflage over the guns and along the roads. In summer, it is not so good, perhaps, as the horizon-blue of the *poilus*, or the green-grey of the Germans, however.

What a picture the French troops made when they drilled! The blue uniforms on the yellow sands, the grey sea and sky beyond, the red sun sinking to the horizon. The English no longer occupied this section, which was given over entirely to the Belgians, with French reserves quartered among the dunes. The moonlight nights at La Panne were too heavenly, the air clear and cold, the sea glorious.

But the Allies do not like moonlight. They no longer sing about "*la belle Lune.*" Instead, they call her the "*Boche lune,*" and "*la sale,*" the dirty, because it is only when she is shining that the Germans come flying over with their deadly bombs. They used to come in the daytime, too, in a different sort of plane that did not carry bombs, but observers with cameras to take photographs. You could see the little white puffs from the anti-aircraft guns curling about them in the blue sky.

The hydro-aeroplane of the Allies looked like huge Silver King tarpon jumping out of the sea, and sometimes they flew so low over the houses that I could tell by the colours on their tails whether they were French, or British, or Belgian.

The noises of La Panne linger in my memory, too—the burr of the *avions*, the tramp of the soldiers, and the bugle calls. Here is one of the calls that used to wake me In the early morning:—

These were the gay sounds, or at least, the cheerful ones. Of another sort were the moaning of the bell buoy and the heart-rending cries from men having their wounds dressed in the operating-room. And then—there was the roar of the big guns.

Naturally, with my work, I did not have time for many walks. Besides, you could not go far without being questioned by guards. But one day, Madame H., who had been there a long time, took me out with her for a stroll.

Perched on a sand dune at the end of the main street was an ugly, forlorn little brown wooden chapel, the Catholic church of La Panne. Mounting the many steps to the door, we entered a cold, empty, pitchy-black place, with one dim candle burning on the altar at the farther end. When my eyes had become more accustomed to the darkness, I saw a solitary soldier standing with bowed head by the railing, and knew that it must have been he who had brought and lighted that one candle for a brother or a comrade fallen in the trenches.

On another dune nearby was a grave, all by itself, with a railing around it. Marking it were a wooden cross and a wreath of black flowers. Here, beneath the white sand, overlooking the dunes and the grey sea, lay one of the bravest and finest women I have ever known— Madame Depage, the doctor's wife. She had worked with him in the Balkan War, and had organised and opened for him the great hospital here. Afterward, she went to America to raise money for their work, and when on her way home was lost on the *Lusitania*. Her body was recovered and laid at rest in this quiet spot.

My companion, Madame H., wished to visit a little military cemetery nearby, where her nephew had been buried. Here there were small black wooden crosses with white letters painted on them— "*Mart pour la patrie*"—and usually a wreath of black tin with bright-coloured flowers of beads or porcelain. Always before I had thought such wreaths hideous beyond words, but somehow here on the sand, in the sunshine, they looked very pretty and cheerful. One of the graves had a photograph of a nice-looking boy at the foot of the mound. A general was there overseeing the arrangements for the funeral of one of his majors who had been killed while handling a "dub." This little cemetery of white sand, looking out over the blue sea, seemed to me an ideal place to rest, it was so clean and pure, and the view so lovely.

There was one other church besides that I have already mentioned, an Episcopal chapel. It was a neat little white building set up on a green lot in the town, evidently built for the British when they were occupying this part of the country, as there was a sign of welcome for the Tommies on the door. It was very bright and cheerful, but rather bare, and seldom used, except by American and English nurses.

We stopped to see the big villa on the beach, where the king and queen had lived when they first came to La Panne. Later, when the British made the place their headquarters, the royal family moved out of the town into Villa Flora, where I had dined with them.

It was a heavenly afternoon, and we wandered about among the dunes with their clumps of scrub, stumbling across some anti-aircraft guns and cannon so marvellously camouflaged in sand houses covered with greens that we did not see them till we were right upon them. Up and down the hills we went, looking here and there into new quarters that were being dug by French reserves.

These, like the shelters for the guns, were scooped out from the side of the mounds, given tin roofs and covered with branches, and sand-bag entrances. These little dwellings looked very homelike and attractive this bright day. Washing fluttered on the bushes, and horses were tethered nearby. It made me long for a taste of the open life myself, and I felt sure that I would like to be a soldier—that is, if I could be a soldier in the dunes.

I think it was Madame H. who told me about those real dwellers in the open, the *Buschkanters*, the Belgian gypsies who had lived for centuries in the woods of West Flanders, and who had only recently been driven from their freeholds by the war. They were a wild, lawless people, living as they pleased and paying taxes to no one. They used to make brooms for a living, and travel all over Europe selling their wares. Now they are scattered forever, and their forest is gone.

In the town we met a couple of officers who looked like Japanese in Belgian uniforms. We made inquiries about them afterward. To my surprise, for I thought I had lived in the East long enough to recognise the different nationalities, they turned out to be two distinguished Chinese officers in the new Chinese uniform, which is almost exactly like the Belgian. Evidently, I have been away from the Far East long enough to lose my eye for Orientals.

An old friend, Colonel D., used to come to dinner quite often at Dr. Depage's, as he was stationed at La Panne, and one night, just before he left, invited the doctor and myself to dine at his mess. He was occupying a small villa not far away, and about a dozen of us sat at the table. I was the only woman present, and except for one French liaison officer, they were all Belgians, so I had to talk French constantly. Listening was even more of a strain than talking, though, because the conversation was interesting, and I did not want to miss anything. They talked very freely before me, and were so kind that I soon felt quite at home among them all.

I took off my cuff and passed it round the table for autographs. It came back with all sorts of things scribbled on it—"The happy wounded!" "No laundry can wash out my love!" "A cuff on the wrist is better than one on the ear." One of the men who had been an artist, made a sketch of an *infirmière*, while another, a musician, wrote a bar of music. Afterward, Dr. Depage and I walked home in the darkness, with the aid of our torchlights.

Another night we were invited to dine with a French general just over the border from Belgium Libre, and to go to a performance given for the *chasseurs*—the "Blue Devils"—who were quartered there at that time. Several of us motored over to a great barn of a house with so many smells about it that I thought we must have struck a factory. But inside there was a homelike sitting-room, and a charming *aide* who assured us that the general would be there at once.

He turned out to be an elderly man, both jovial and polite. A major who had just come from Paris sat next to me, and I asked him many questions about the latest news. On the front one feels out of the world, as one sees only local newspapers and knows nothing of what is going on outside his particular section.

After dinner we all got into motors and drove off—I do not know where—and came to a stop under the spire of a church with a big full moon behind it. There was a walk through pitch-black alleyways. At the end of one, seemingly out of the blackness, came shouts of laughter. A small door opened somewhere, and we went into a huge hall, crowded with *chasseurs*. These are the shock troops, and they had won the *fourragère* or cord over the shoulder, showing that the whole regiment had been exceptionally brave. Most of the men had been decorated besides. They looked very jaunty with their little tarns, or *bérets*, and their navy-blue uniforms.

I sat beside a one-armed general with steely blue eyes and grey hair. On the other side was their *commandant*, a huge man, with a handsome set of false teeth (he had evidently been wounded in the mouth), who wore endless decorations. He enjoyed the performance immensely, waving to the leading actress, whom he seemed to know very well.

While the moon was full, we kept wondering if the Boche *avions* would come, and what they would do to La Panne. They had not entirely forgotten it in the past, as several demolished houses in the village testified, but while they generally flew over on their way to and from England, they seemed not to think it worthwhile to waste their ammunition on so small a place and on a hospital, and generally saved their compliments for Dunkirk and Calais.

But this time they thought differently, or wanted a change, perhaps. We were just finishing dinner one night when we heard the anti-aircraft guns. I ran to the window and saw, over the sands, star lights dropping in the sky, and sparks from shrapnel, and heard the loud bangs of exploding bombs. Most of these fell round Adinkerke, however, a couple of miles to the south.

One day sixty entrants came into the hospital from the town itself—not victims of German bombs or long-range guns, but of some Belgian hand grenades exploding in a house filled with soldiers. Nobody ever discovered exactly what happened. Soldiers who arrived that morning had put the grenades in the cellar, although it was against military rules to keep them in a building where troops were quartered. An old couple lived in the basement of the house, and it was thought the grenades might have been left too near the stove—at least, that was the theory advanced by a man who came into the operating room with a broken arm. He was just outside when it occurred—there was a frightful explosion, and half the house fell, covering him with debris.

I shall never forget the sight of the wounded hobbling down the street, trying to stumble along by themselves, or leaning on their comrades, bleeding, dusty, and with torn clothes; others were on stretchers, or in ambulances, or borne in the arms of fellow soldiers.

I went that afternoon to interview the old couple who had lived in the basement. Grey, bent and withered, they were standing dejectedly among the ruins of their home. The door had been blown off, and all about them were scattered broken furniture and dishes. Both were so dazed by the sudden catastrophe that they could tell little of what had happened, and that only in Flemish. The old man had been just about to open the cellar door to get some potatoes, when his wife spoke to him and he was delayed. If he had gone when he intended, he would have been killed. As it was, they lost all they had in the world, and had no place to sleep.

People began to talk about the spring drive. Guns were mysteriously put up among the villas. The Boches were most anxious to get Nieuport, to the north of us, for that controlled the flooded district which was so important a means of defence for the Allies. It was expected, too, that they would make another try for Ypres, in order to get through to Calais.

But wherever I went, the people were sure their section would be attacked first. While I was working at Épernay, the feeling was that the Boches would come through the valley of the Marne during their next drive, as they had done so successfully in 1914. When the British came to Cugny and the French moved out, it was thought something would

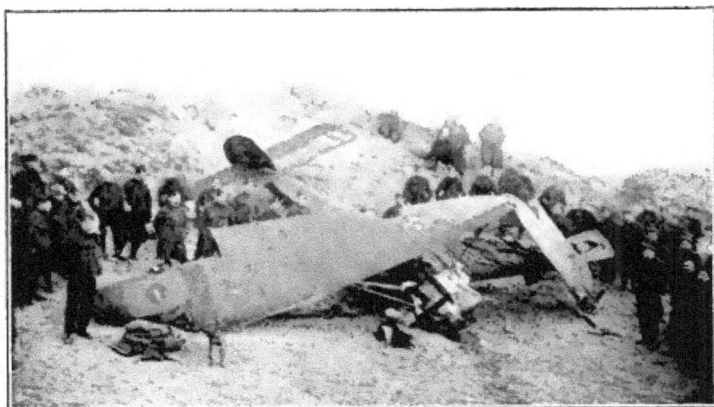

CAPTAIN DEPAGE'S FALLEN PLANE

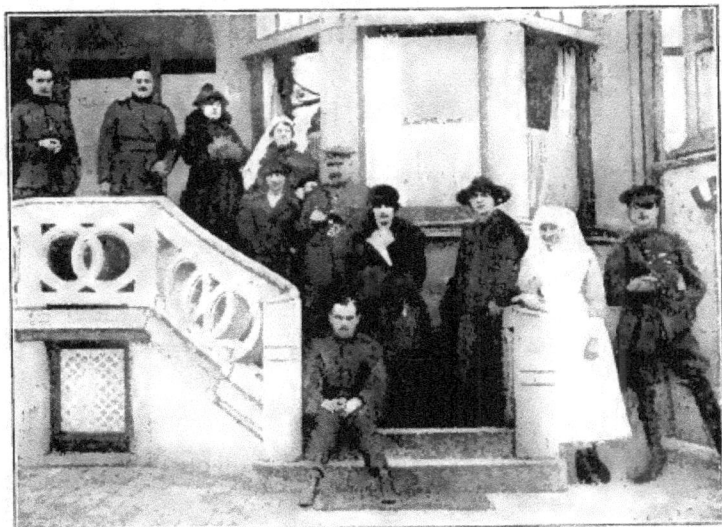

AT LA PANNE, FEBRUARY 15, 1918
Left to right: 2d, Dr. Vandervelde; 4th, Mrs. Anderson; 6th, Dr. Depage;
seated, Captain Depage

be doing, because as a rule the Britishers made attacks and stirred things up, and the Boches were especially fond of going for them.

When the spring offensive actually did begin, in the north, it looked as if the whole Belgian Army was on the move. I never saw better marching. Bands passed along the beach, and trumpet calls blew all day long. Line after line of troops went by, headed by officers on horseback, and dashing cavalry. It was no mere parade, for in one day a hundred wounded came in to our hospital from Merckem.

We had news one night that the flying machine of Dr. Depage's son had been shot down. But fortunately, the boy had not even been hurt. He brought the pilot to dine with us, and they told of their thrilling escape. Their *avion* had twenty-nine holes in it, and the pilot almost lost control, so they came swooping down into the sand dunes at a terrific rate. Why they were not both killed, no one knows.

Young Depage had done excellent work in the past, taking photographs beyond the lines, and several times he had been recommended for bravery. We were not especially surprised, but of course much delighted, when his *Croix de Guerre* arrived. He was a nice, well set up, attractive lad, at this time a captain in the aviation corps, though he had served in the Belgian Army before.

We had luncheon with Captain Depage one day at the Belgian aviation camp. The quarters were in temporary buildings near an old farm. There were tables at one end of the main room for reading and writing, and small dinner tables at the other end. We lunched with the handsome young officer who was in command, having an omelette, ham, American pickles, beef, potatoes, oranges, and red wine. Another barrack had been divided off into small bedrooms. Captain Depage had made his attractive with bright chintzes and pictures.

Outside, we inspected the hangars for the flying machines—great flapping tents of canvas, all camouflaged. I saw the aeroplane guns, and some photographs taken at great heights, which showed the straight lines of the roads and railways and canals, and the winding ones of the rivers, and also towns that had been demolished, and holes made by *obus*. The Belgians, I hear, take the very best photographs from aeroplanes.

They told me the queen was very fond of going up in the *avions*, and that she had actually flown back over the enemy's lines till she could look down on the villages and fields of the country from which she had been an exile so long. The king, too, went over frequently, I understood. They have even flown across the Channel.

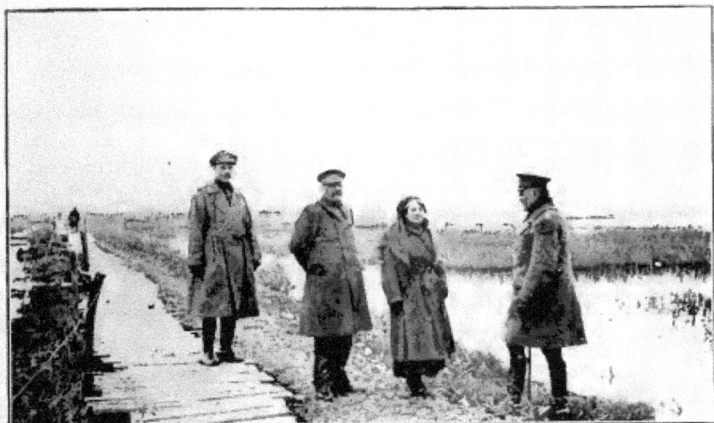

BEYOND THE FRONT-LINE TRENCHES BETWEEN NIEUPORT
AND PERVYSE

Left to right: Lieutenant de Young, General Drubbel, Mrs. Anderson,
Captain Cresson

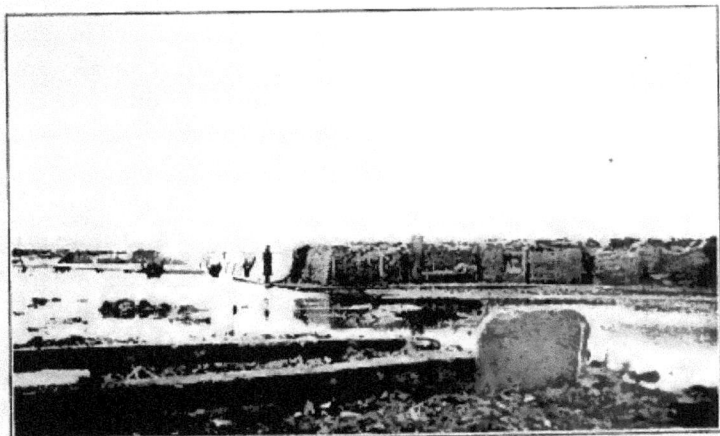

FERME LA VEUVE

Thanks to Captain Cresson, our American liaison officer, I had another trip to the trenches. We passed on the way the *château* where the Minister of War, M. de Koeninck, the only minister at the front, was living. At last we came to a farmhouse. It was the usual farm, with chickens and ducks all about, and the usual dirty pool of water in the middle of the courtyard. Captain Cresson knocked at the door and an orderly ushered us into a bare room whose walls were hung with maps.

General Drubbel, who had been in the war from the beginning, was sitting behind a table littered with papers. He gave us a cordial welcome, and drove with us out to Avecapelle, a little town with only a few houses and part of a church left standing. There in a patched-up house he proudly showed us one of his "libraries." It was one of several, he explained, that he was starting for the use of his troops, because he felt that in spite of the fact that the towns were being constantly bombarded, a place for the men to read was a necessity.

It was a pathetic little library, it had so few books, and no writing-paper at all, and the fire was lighted only in the afternoon. I promised to get magazines and writing-paper for him. Just in front of the house was a big *obus* hole, made the afternoon before by a shell which fortunately did not explode and was buried and left there. That same day, another shell had hit the already half-demolished church.

After stopping a moment at a small portable house which proved to be a fencing club for officers, we returned to the farmhouse headquarters for luncheon. The small room was crowded. The general, who was very jolly, introduced the officers and asked me to sit opposite him. The meal was a lively one. We drank each other's healths in American champagne and had many jokes about the favourite subject of *marraines*.

After luncheon the general and one of his *aides*, Captain de Young, took us to see a unique review. It was nothing less than a corps of dogs, some thirty in all, hauling guns! They were doing the best work of any dogs in the war, and the general was as proud of them as he was of his libraries.

They were of indescribable breed, some like St. Bernards, others plain mongrels. They might have been the same animals that drew milk carts through city streets in the days of peace, but war had given them added virtues, for they no longer barked, and would do all manner of things at command. A gun, mounted on wheels, was pulled by two dogs, and accompanied by two men. It was quite a sight to see them dragging their guns along, turning this way or that as directed by their masters. The general said that their success depended largely on their trainers. When off duty the dogs were kept near together, living in small wooden kennels grouped in pairs, with pointed roofs. Their diet consisted of bread, water, and meat. Although bad roads were hard on their paws, they could travel much farther in a day than a man. On the whole, dogs have not proved a success in the war. This was the one corps that had done splendid service.

Speaking of dogs, I was told that candidates for the British canine military service had to undergo a rigid physical examination before a jury of experts. Those accepted were taken "for duration" and sent to centres of instruction, where they were taught the soldierly virtues of courage, prudence, and discipline. After a long course under experienced trainers, they were sent to the front. The Blue Cross established hospitals for them, which "moved with the army," each one having a veterinary surgeon and several attendants to care for the ill or wounded dogs.

From the review we were hurried on to Ramscapelle, and I was especially fortunate in going there with the general, for it was in this historic spot that he took his great stand with the *Zouaves* and turned back the Germans in 1914. The village was quite destroyed, but even while we walked there among the ruins it was under fire.

Then we skirted the railroad line only a few yards away from the first-line trenches. It was a quiet day, and the guns were not nearly so lively as on the afternoon I went into the trenches south of Dixmude. Besides, this was in the flooded district and we felt quite safe behind the camouflage of the road. Occasionally, a Boche shell would whiz by over our heads, and there were endless *obus* holes all about.

On one side of the road were scattered little huts, where the cooking for the troops was done, and first-aid stations. On the other side was the camouflage of leafless bushes which hid both the road and the huts from the enemy lying in wait beyond the expanse of shallow, muddy water with its tufts of yellow grass sticking up here and there,

I was glad to see what the inside of one of these army dressing-stations was like. This was very primitive, consisting of a couple of cellar rooms. In one of these the doctor slept; the other, for the wounded, was empty except for its stretchers, bandages, and few bottles, and was kept very clean. The doctor showed me with great pride his new gas mask, in which he could work during a gas attack. It seemed quite elaborate after the simple ones we were given.

At a hole in the camouflage screen, some distance farther on, we got out of the motor and went through on a board walk about a quarter of a mile, till we came to the huts of the first-line trenches, so called, though they weren't exactly that because there were outposts of men and guns beyond, on islands in the inundated land. These outposts were reached by stepping stones, and were so well hidden among bushes that we could not see them.

The general took us out on the plank walk beyond the trenches into the water. Knowing nothing about it, it did seem rather risky to me, but I suppose he knew whether it was comparatively safe. Anyway, we stopped and had our photographs taken there. The water was what remained of the flood which poured in when the dykes were opened, in 1914, and prevented the Boches from reaching Calais.

The trenches were much like those I have already described by the river—a wall of mud and earth overgrown by grass, with small living quarters made solid by sand bags.

Just behind the lines nearby was Pervyse, a village without a house left standing. But over a cellar waved a flag with a red cross. There lived those two brave British women, Mrs. Knocker, now Baroness de T'Serclaes, and Miss Chisholm, of whom so much has been written. One is Scotch, the other English, and both young and extremely good-looking. (*Vide The Cellar-House of Pervyse* by G. E. Mitton, the true story about long-time friends and motorcycling companions, widow Elsie 'Gypsy' Knocker and Mairi Chisholm; Leonaur, 2011.) They wore khaki uniforms—high boots and breeches, long coats, and brown silk veils.

The women showed us the three rooms of their tiny cellar house— their sitting-room, with a fire, a small, dark hole with two bunks where they slept, and a place for first aid. In September, 1914, they had gone to Belgium as nurses, retreating from Ghent as the Germans came on, but taking their stand here in Pervyse three months later, and remaining through thick and thin. Nobody knows how much they have done for the soldiers of Belgium, with their skilled hands and cheerful faces. It has been a wonderful work, carried out in spite of every sort of danger and handicap.

I wish that we might have had more time to talk with them. They offered us tea, and asked after a soldier whom they had sent to Ocean Hospital that morning with a bullet wound in his head, and then we had to go on our way again.

During the spring drive, the fighting became intense around Pervyse, and both women were gassed. When I went through London,

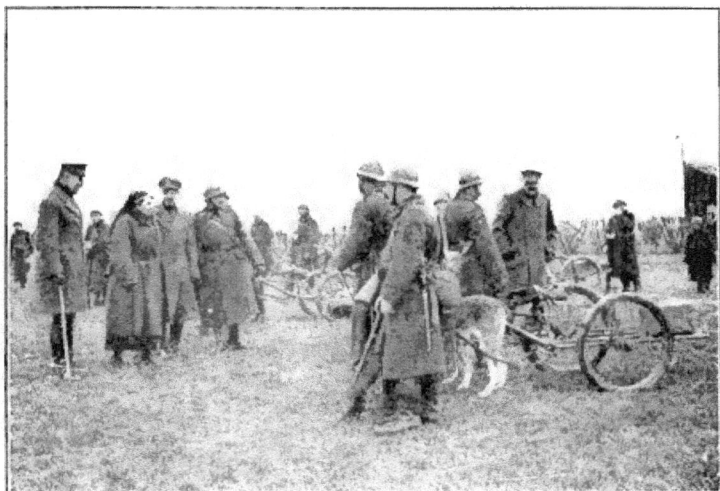

BELGIAN WAR DOGS

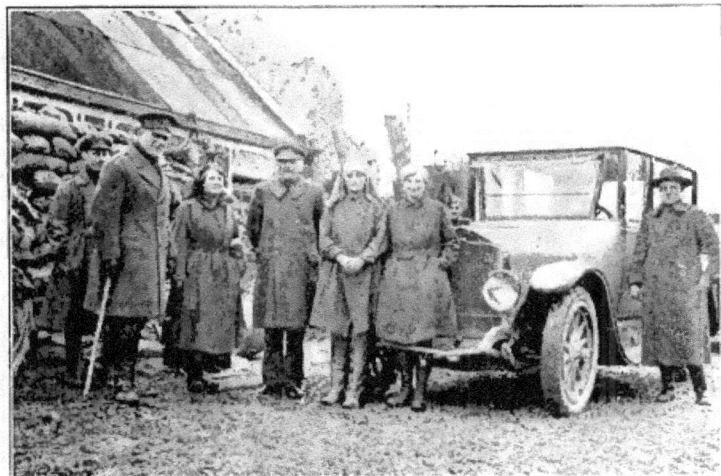

BEFORE THE CELLAR HOUSE AT PERVYSE
Left to right: Lieutenant de Young, Captain Cresson, Mrs. Anderson, General
Drubbel, Baroness de T'Serclaes, Miss Chisholm

I heard they were in a hospital there, recovering, and that they were moving heaven and earth for permission to go back to their post. But the British Government refused to let them go, because they said it was too dangerous. I can't understand why a woman has not just as much right to die for her country as a man, if she wants to.

At the cross-roads near Pervyse we climbed up into a demolished cemetery with open, gaping graves, because it was on higher ground and we could get a better view. While we were having our pictures taken there, two army wagons appeared. The general had the drivers included in the picture, asked their names and addresses, and said he would send them prints. No wonder he is popular with his troops!

As it was getting late and time to return to headquarters, we made our way back past the barbed wire and unused trenches, our car swaying in the muddy ruts of the road. We said goodbye to the jolly, brave old officer and his young lieutenant and set off toward home.

But our day was not yet over, for Captain Cresson and I stopped at a canteen near Furnes, kept by two English women. It was larger and more comfortable than the one at Loo, and was made gay with flowers. Some Belgian officers were having tea when we went in. These two women, the two at Pervyse, and the one at Loo, are the only women who have special permits from the king to work so near the lines in Belgium, and I do not know of any who are allowed to do this sort of thing in France.

Very different was an army canteen operated by a soldier for the general's division. It gave out hot coffee, to be sure, but was really more of a store where the men could buy things at low cost. I tried some of this coffee myself, and at the time thought it was very good, but since coming home I realise that I did not have a good cup of coffee in my entire eight months' absence!

CHAPTER 8

Ocean Hospital

Vous ne reverrez plus les monts, les bois, la terre,
Beaux yeux de mes soldats qui n'aviez que vingt ans
Et qui êtes tombés, en ce dernier printemps,
Où plus que jamais douce apparut la lumière.

The following notes are taken from my journal:—

"I am sitting on the radiator pipes in the corner of the operating-room, not to keep warm, for of course the operating-room is always tropical, but because there are no chairs. For the moment there is nothing going on. I have finished my work of putting Vaseline and gauze in a tin box to be sterilised and am simply on duty.

"There is so much to write about when I do have a minute to myself that I don't know where to begin. Just looking out of the window here I see going past a French officer on horseback, two sailors afoot, a Belgian trumpeter, a blind soldier led by a man with one eye, a patient without legs having his turn out of doors in a basket wagon on wheels, an English motorcyclist; the king's motor, a two-wheeled market cart, an ambulance; bandaged heads and limping legs, steel helmet and soft cap, gas mask and *sabot*; overhead an ever-present flying machine.

"The uniforms make the streets look gay, in spite of the many things which are sad to see. High boots and brown caps with a red or silver tassel swinging from the front upper point and the high standing collar with colour are characteristic of the Belgian soldiers. The British you can tell at once by the low collar, and the Americans by the high collar without colour, but their khaki uniforms in the distance look somewhat alike. I find the insignia of rank in the different armies rather perplexing. Both French and Belgian doctors have red velvet

97

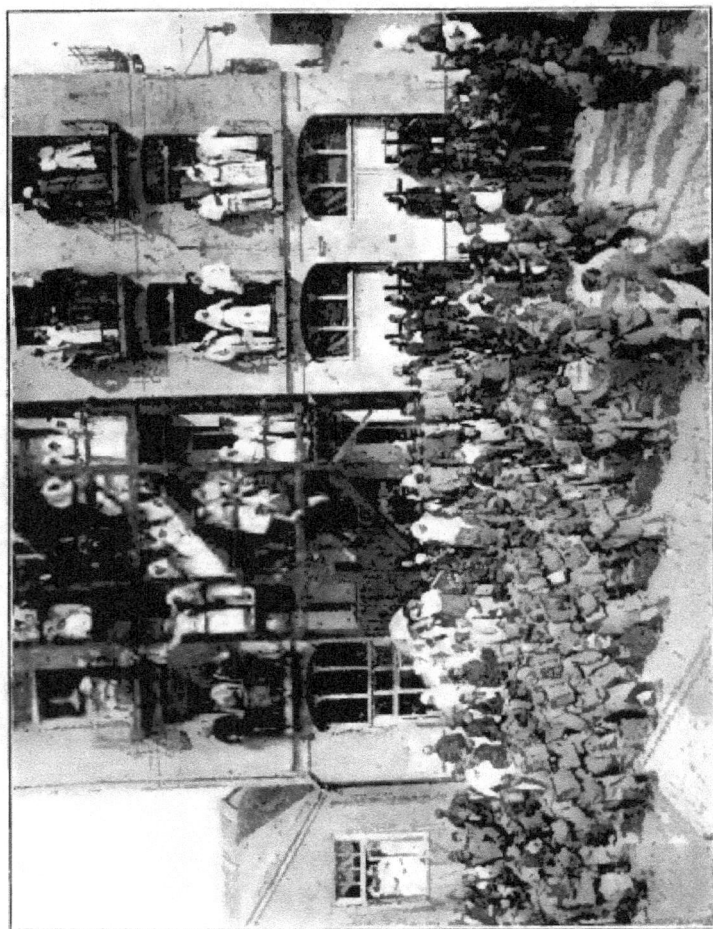

OCEAN HOSPITAL

collars so they can be easily distinguished.

"An ambulance has just drawn up at the door of the receiving-room. I sigh and say, 'Poor devil!' The flap at the back is carefully opened and out comes—the hospital wash!

"Here in this operating-room, which is principally for fractures, there are three operating-tables and several long tables with endless bottles—alcohol, ether and Dakin solution are those most in demand—and shining instruments all beautifully laid out and sterilised, of course, and covered up with a sheet. (I have worked here so long now that even when I am off duty, I hardly feel that I can touch anything without pincers!) In round tin boxes are sterilised towels and pads, cotton-wool balls, and compresses. These are all necessary, for most of the wounds have Carrel tubes and need the pads to soak up the moisture.

"I have spent hours preparing those Carrel tubes, cutting the rubber tubing and puncturing them with small holes—some with a few, some with many—and tying them at the end with a string. The theory is that to keep a wound thoroughly disinfected, it must be kept moist with Dakin solution, which is done in this way: In the wards, a tube in the wound is attached to another which is put on a glass bottle and hung at the top of the bed. Every two hours, the nurse on duty opens the metal clasp on the long tube and counts four, watching carefully to make sure the solution is flowing as it should, then closing the clasp again. The Carrel treatment with the Dakin solution is used at all the hospitals over here. There are other solutions used in certain cases, such as flavine and brilliant green, but the Carrel treatment is employed much more commonly and with great success.

"Dr. Depage put me here in the *salle* where wounds are dressed and operations performed. I work under Dr. Vandervelde, with three charming Belgian nurses who are very nice to me. At first, I merely dusted and prepared the tables, and rolled long strips of gauze for plaster casts, and washed the instruments, and got the rubber gloves and the bowls ready to be sterilized, but before long I was waiting on the doctors, buttoning on their white operating coats, handing them sterilized articles with pincers, filling ether bottles, covering ether masks, blowing white powder on stumps, holding irrigation jars, cutting off old bandages, and even bandaging up wounds.

"I have gradually gotten into the doctors' ways, and so now know exactly what they want for certain types of wounds and have everything ready for them without their asking.

"The only things which I have not done that all experienced nurses do is to shave the men (which apparently is not difficult, but there has never been time to learn) and to give the anaesthetics. The girls offered to teach me this, but I did not wish to kill anyone, and we were so very busy that I said we would wait for a quiet moment. That moment has never come, and probably never will, for we seem always busy.

"Such terrible wounds as we see here in this *salle!* Almost every man has an arm or a leg gone, or a bad wound in the back or thigh, and they often have all one side injured. One man has a leg so mangled that you can look quite through it in two places. I really don't see how he can live, but they say he will.

"A fine blond Flemish soldier was hurried to us direct from the trenches without being even cleaned, because he needed to be operated on at once. He had been wounded at three in the morning, but did not reach us until eleven. The Germans had taken the trench and not wishing to bother with him had left him to die, but the Belgians recaptured the trench and sent him back. The doctor had to cut off both his legs, as both were badly smashed and gangrene had begun to set in. The amputating is done very quickly. A knife is used first, then a sharpened saw. When a leg drops off into the pail with a thud it gives me a shock, for it stands upright instead of crumpling up and collapsing, as I somehow feel it should when it is no longer a part of the body.

"The other day a man died on the operating table—he had a bad stump already cut very short. It was in such a terrible condition from gangrene that I was almost glad when he could die, poor man, so peacefully, asleep under the ether.

"I don't see how these Belgian nurses, so young and pretty, are able to stand the dreadful sights and do their work so well.

"The other day, when I was bandaging the stump of a soldier's right arm, he said to me so sweetly in French 'I am lucky to have one hand. Yes, I believe I can work with that.' His left arm was injured, too, but I think will come out all right. A soldier who had both legs cut off and a wound in his head besides is doing very well. It is wonderful how brave they are. Among the wounded here we have two brothers, both struck by the same shell.

"A hundred *entrants* came in today, for the drive has begun, in this region at any rate. Ambulances go whizzing past the operating *salle* (which, by the way, is in a portable tin house with the imposing name of Albert and Elisabeth Hall) to the door of the receiving-room near-by. A few soldiers and *infirmières* gather about them, and the *brancardiers* lift out stretchers bearing limp forms covered with dark blankets.

"The fighting is getting lively near Dixmude. The roar of the guns from Nieuport was very heavy last night. I spent the evening in the hall here in the hospital, listening to an excellent concert—or to what I could hear of it. An attack must have been going on, for the cannon were so loud that the house shook, and it was hard to listen to the music. I couldn't help wondering why we were sitting there so calmly and doing nothing when perhaps at that very moment the Boches were dashing down upon us.

"But after the concert was over, I walked home alone as usual in the blackness and crept up the three flights of dark stairs to my little corner, where I boiled some water and had a drink of malted milk, grabbed my hot-water bottle, and tumbled into bed all dressed—not because I was afraid of the Boches, but to keep warm.

"I wonder if we shall ever have to spend our nights in those zig-zag, sand-bagged trenches, with a tin cover at one end, down on the beach in front of the house, and if the barbed wire there will be a real protection?

"The whistle for a gas attack has gone off twice lately, but nobody seemed to bother about it—perhaps it was a false alarm. I saw an officer just back from the front who had been in a very bad gas attack, from which many had died on the field. His description was not pleasant.

"To change the subject—there is a delightful little clubhouse for the nurses which is called 'The Clock,' and looks like a Dutch doll house. (About a week after I left La Panne this tea house was completely destroyed, by a bomb, but no one was killed. See Appendix.) We go there and have tea with sugar, and bread, milk and butter, all free. We toast the bread ourselves and take jam and cake with us.

"It gives us a nice chance to rest and talk over the news. A few letters have come out from Brussels lately with bad tidings. They say there is very little bread there, and everybody is weak from lack of nourishment. The Germans have made a systematic search of every house and taken all the mattresses and blankets.

"Speaking of Brussels, a most extraordinary story was told me the other day, and I saw the man to whom it happened, a pale, slight fellow, very distinguished-looking. He had flown to Brussels, circled about the house of his parents, from whom he had heard nothing for a long time, and dropped a letter with news of himself. They recognised him and waved. He flew back to La Panne and reported what he had done, a most daring and unheard-of performance. Of course, he had had no orders to do such a thing, and so instead of at least receiving the *Croix de Guerre*, he was given eight days in the guard-house.

"Last night we heard that a Pole who had been fighting with the Boches came over to the Belgians and gave them much information. But unfortunately, a Belgian also went over to the Boches.

"Sometimes I write in a small room off the operating-room, at a table where a little alcohol lamp is always burning, near two gas-jets over which we boil the instruments. On one side is the sink, on the other a glass cupboard filled with shining, strange-looking instruments and lots of little bundles that contain sterilized rubber gloves for the doctors, marked with the different sizes. Below, the catgut and morphine and various things are kept. There is another large cupboard of white tin boxes with the Red Cross on them which contain every known article for hospital use, from safety pins to bandages—even splints and old bones.

"In an adjoining room the *brancardiers* work. During the afternoon they have little to do. One of them, a Walloon named Julien, studies, for he is trying to learn to read and write. The other two are both Flemish. Julien confided to me that before the war he was a gardener and grew rare orchids. After being wounded twice in the army, he had been taken into the hospital to work, and he said he liked it here so much that he thought after the war he would remain. Unless, he added, his wife, who was in Brussels, joined him and was willing to go with him to America.

"Dr. Vandervelde is away just now, and Dr. Depage operates almost daily, generally putting in plates to connect broken bones. The patient is put under ether and a long slit is made. The most trying part is putting the screws in the plate to hold the bones; the screws do not always fit, and sometimes break, and it seems to require a lot of strength to get them in. The huge, powerful figure of the doctor, in his spectacles and his long white operating coat, with the sweat rolling down his forehead, looks something like an intellectual but thoroughly angry suffragette.

"With a *brancardier* holding the electric light, and with nurses and visiting doctors, we make a group of ten at least. As the blood spatters over the white sheets and drips on the floor, it makes a picture that I don't believe I shall ever forget.

"The British, I understand, do not altogether approve of this method of plating. They say it is all very well for the surgeons at the front to do it, but months later in the base hospitals a great many plates have to be taken out before the wounds heal, so they believe in grafting the bone and not moving the fractured limb till the process is completed. If the limb is plated, it can be moved much sooner, of course—in fact, such cases are brought into the dressing-room every day in this hospital, while in the British hospitals they are kept in bed. We have a general here who had broken his leg, but he was allowed to go about in an amazingly short time and seems to be doing nicely.

"There are moments when I am a little tired of getting up at dawn and preparing my own breakfast in a stone-cold room, where my fingers are so numb, I can hardly hold the dishes. What is wanted over here is simply women who have strong arms and legs—you should be young and well and willing to do what you are told. The heads of departments are few and naturally they are women who have been working since the beginning of the war and intend to work until the end, not people who have only signed up for six months or so.

"While I was sitting in 'The Clock' this afternoon word came for me to go to Dr. Depage's house. Opening the glass doors to the dining-room, whom should I see sitting at the table, but the queen! She got up and shook hands, and the doctor asked me to have chocolate with them.

"Her Majesty wore a white cloth suit and a simple white hat. She asked if my husband was angry because she had let me go into the trenches, and wanted to know how it happened that the French had let me off to come and work in Belgium. Of course, I explained that I was working in my *permission*. She smoked a cigarette and chatted very pleasantly with us. When I was in Brussels, before the war, none of the ladies smoked, but now they all do. '*C'est la guerre!*'

"Dr. V., who had come in, remarked that he occasionally smoked a pipe, and Her Majesty said the king did, too, sometimes, and she often cleaned his pipe for him, but feared she didn't do it very well. It seems they had just come back from a trip, and she told Dr. V. that she wanted to begin work again in his operating-room.

"The queen arrived at ten o'clock this morning, and stayed for two hours. We had given the *salle* an extra cleaning and got a special outfit all ready for Her Majesty—the usual white rubber apron and white cotton overshoes and rubber gloves. Instead of the white veil which French and Belgian nurses wear, she put on a sort of turban cap of white silk.

"She came in very quietly, and we all curtsied. Then, as she dressed the wounds, doing the work of the doctors, we waited upon her. I stood behind the movable table with dressings. Her first case was a man with a very bad arm, her second a man who had both legs cut off. She used to do this sort of thing in hospitals even before the war.

"I think it is quite wonderful of her to work so hard, and to do it so well. For it is not pleasant to see such dreadful wounds, all open and bleeding, and to hear men groaning and grinding their teeth with pain, some crying and yelling and biting their blankets, and, when under the influence of ether, talking so strangely.

"When she is through, the nurses take turns helping her off with her gloves and overshoes, and as she goes out, we all curtsy again. This noon, after she had gone, I went into the *brancardiers'* room and found Julien greatly enjoying himself, imitating the way we curtsied to the queen. We have had other royal visitors—among them the Queen of England's brother, the Prince of Teck. He often comes to inquire about men in whom he is interested, for although the hospital is principally filled with Belgians, we also have some wounded Tommies. As I knew the British doctor who accompanies the prince, in Wimereux, he asked me one day to join them on their round and tell His Highness about the patients. The prince, a big, handsome man, with a pleasant word for all, reminded me in many ways of King Albert."

CHAPTER 9

Belgium Libre

Belgium Libre, the part of Belgium left to the king, is very small. The northern boundary runs along the railway and canal from Nieuport, near the many "*capelles*" and the much-fought-over Dixmude and Ypres to the French frontier. In all, it is a territory some ten miles wide by thirty long, but its size varies from day to day according to the trenches that are taken or lost. There is not a single square yard of it that cannot be reached by enemy fire. Scattered here and there along the front are farms now inhabited by Belgian soldiers, and demolished villages, while behind are more thickly populated towns. But the whole civilian population is less than a hundred thousand.

This Belgium of today (1918) is a small part of what used to be West Flanders, and the people are Flemish—a stolid folk whose methods of farming and indeed of everything are those of a century ago. In from the sea, the country is flat and unattractive. Along the roads the poplars are all bent one way by the wind, and the willow stumps look like worn-out feather dusters. Occasionally there is a windmill or a glimpse of sand dunes and blue sea, with small boats out after shrimp.

The king is commander of the Belgian Army, about two hundred thousand in number. They are men who have suffered everything and have nothing left to lose but their lives. Homes, families, they have none. So, they keep guard over their heroic king and queen and the pitiful remnant of their country with a faithfulness and loyalty that to my mind is almost mediaeval. Even under these distressing circumstances, the army has increased, for before the war it was only half its present size.

During the spring attack this appeared in a British paper:—

The behaviour of the Belgian troops seems to have been magnificent. They went into counter-attack singing. Officers could not find words to describe the enthusiasm with which the men threw themselves into battle. The Belgian artillery is said to have been very good. Belgian aviators flew so low over the German positions, machine gunning as they flew, that their machines were spattered with mud from the shells exploding in the soft ground below. The infantry on the ground cheered and saluted the aviators overhead. A really splendid spirit seems to have pervaded all arms engaged. The news of the victory was received with exultation and rejoicing throughout the Belgian Army, and both British and French are immensely proud of their allies. Individual Belgians of all ranks appear to have fought like men possessed, utterly regardless of self and full of fury and contempt for the enemy. (See Appendix.)

In striking contrast to the soldiers are the *flamingants*, or activists, who are the product of ignorance and German propaganda. They are like our I.W.W.'s, the Irish rebels, and the pacifists; most of them are uneducated and do not understand the situation or know what they are talking about. They are ruled by their priests, who, like those in Ireland, Canada, and Australia, have made so much trouble for the Allies. (And yet, some of the heroes of Belgium have been priests! That is another contrast.) These *flamingants* are such a lawless lot that the civilians have to carry guns to protect themselves against them. Of course, some of them are spies; and the leaders are paid by the Germans.

In order to counteract any influence which the *Flamingint* movement may have, King Albert goes out and talks to the troops, praising and encouraging them. The king is fine and big and intelligent, a man who reads much and thinks things out for himself, and is brave, too, going constantly into the trenches.

While in La Panne I had many chances to see the varied activities that are being carried on in this strip of land which five years ago was a forgotten corner of a prosperous country.

Dr. Depage took me one day to his colossal hospital at Winckem, five miles distant. It was planned much like the French *auto-chir* at Cugny, only on a larger and finer scale. The main building, which was of wood, had a corridor half a mile long, with barracks built from it at intervals for the wards, operating-rooms, etc. The kitchen, of yellow brick and architecturally very good, was a separate building, and was equipped with hand-cars to take the food to the patients.

Both last year and this, when the spring drive began, Ocean Hospital had to be evacuated and the patients were sent to Winckem. But even here it was too near the front for safety, and I believe this year the men had to be moved still farther back, even as far as Calais. It was still unfinished when I saw it, owing to the lack of workmen. The English had expected to take over this hospital, but their troops were moved farther south. I believe the doctor's idea is to turn these buildings into an agricultural school after the war, but it would prove useful as a hospital, even when peace comes, because large institutions will be needed for the cripples.

Of a very different sort was the small first operating station of the Belgian Red Cross, to which, through the doctor's kindness, two nurses and myself went in a motor. It was two miles back from the lines—a pretty little pick-up house with tiny bedrooms and a living-room heated by a stove. Opposite was another collapsible building, the most complete little hospital that I ever saw. It had only six beds, and rarely more than half of these were filled, for only abdominal and chest cases that had to be operated on immediately were brought here. There were also several tents to be used for services, as a morgue, and so on. The staff consisted of two doctors, two *infirmières*, and a priest in khaki.

After a delicious little luncheon, we drove on in an ambulance to within a mile of the trenches and saw once more the hidden guns and camouflaged roads and the hay-mounds made into dwellings, besides some bombarded houses patched up with cement and occupied by soldiers. In an old cemetery nearby, quite demolished, was the biggest *obus* hole I had ever seen, made by a shell from a 210 gun. One of the nurses who had come with us from La Panne told me that her husband had been killed on this very road, only three months before.

One morning the queen sent a motor for me and, after getting the matron's permission—you could not move without telling her exactly where you were going, for the rules were very strict—I drove out to Villa Flora. This time it was broad daylight, so there was a chance to see what the outside of the *château* where the king and queen were living really looked like. It was a two-storeyed dwelling, not large, and of good architecture, built of grey brick with many white blinds. There was a small driveway in front, and a farm building opposite.

Countess Van den Steen de Jehay got into the motor, and we drove to the *Maison Militaire du Roi*, a few miles away. This was a big, ugly-looking house where the king's suite were lodged, the officers taking turns in going on duty for two weeks at a time, just as the queen's ladies-in-waiting did.

The count and an officer joined us and we travelled south past Cavour and Beveren, both big hospitals. One of the men explained the derivation of the word Boche, which I had not heard before. At the beginning of the war Albosch, the name of a small part of Germany, was turned into Sale Bosche, *sale* of course meaning dirty, and applied to all Germans. This was finally abbreviated and spelled as it is now—Boche.

On the way we passed a British airplane that had just fallen and lay on its side, like a bird with a broken wing. A crowd of silent soldiers were standing about it, and an ambulance. We did not stop to look any further.

At last the motor arrived at Couthoven, which was one of the small hospitals run by the countess's cousin for the civilian population of this region. It consisted of portable barracks set up in the park of a beautiful *château*. The British were occupying this section, and they had padded the outside of the barracks with earth halfway to the roof in a fashion I had not seen before, making the walls so solid that only a direct hit from a *taube* could demolish them.

The convalescents—all who were able to hobble about—were sitting in the sun that shone down through the trees, or lay on beds which had been brought out for them. Nuns in flapping white head-dresses tended them. It was a picturesque sight, but sad.

Two of the nurses were Americans, but the rest were nuns who had come from Ypres and Poperinghe and gave their services without pay. They were devotion itself, the countess told me, adding that one of their number had been killed by a bomb at her hospital in Poperinghe.

Madame Terlinden, who was working here with the countess, had a little house of her own—two rooms, one for sleeping, the other for living, made cosy with chintz and pictures. She showed me the portraits of her husband and daughter, both prisoners in Germany. Her son was in the army and her daughter-in-law working in the operating-room. Her husband, I believe, had been imprisoned because he had helped Belgians across the border. At his trial a German officer said to the daughter, "I think I have seen you before—you look rather English. Or is it that you look like some English woman whom I have seen?" The girl answered, rather impertinently, "Perhaps I remind you of Miss Cavell." For this she was imprisoned for a month.

A dear old *abbé* came in and had luncheon with us. It was a good

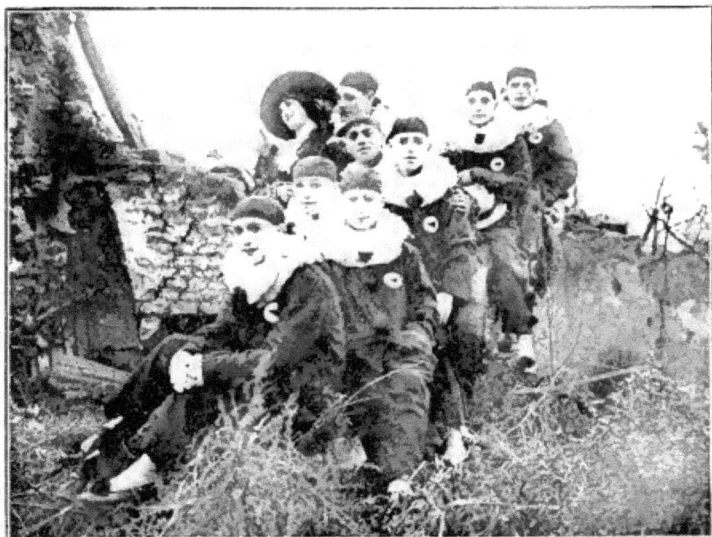

"THE JOCKS," A SCOTCH ENTERTAINMENT TROUPE

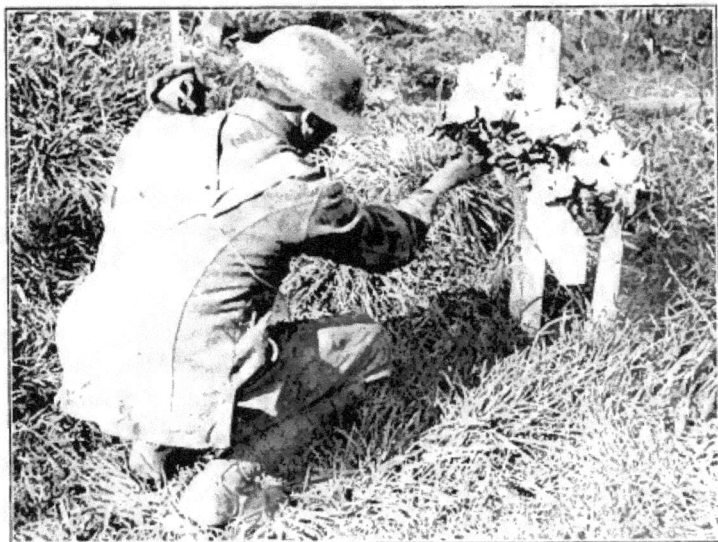

AFTER THE BATTLE OF BROODSEYNDE, NEAR YPRES

luncheon too—beer, beef and bread. It really was surprising what good things the workers had to eat there in Belgium Libre—very different from what the poor Belgians beyond the trenches were getting!

On the way back to La Panne we passed the great British cemetery filled with little white crosses, near Crucifix Corner, named in memory of the heavy fighting there which had cost so many lives. One of the things which had surprised me most in France was to see how few trees had been cut down, but this day we saw the forest of Baron B., surrounding his *château*, going under the axe. I understand that now both French and English are sacrificing their forests.

One of the nurses in our hospital at La Panne, who had been in Japan a few years before, was asked to give a lecture at the big military hospital in Beveren. She took with her some other *infirmières*, who played the piano and violin and sang, and they gave selections from *Madam Butterfly*. Her own lantern slides were excellent, and a Belgian officer who had also been in Japan told amusing stories. The hall was gaily decorated and filled with patients and nurses. The front row was reserved for wounded on stretchers.

It was on this trip we noticed that still more wire defences had been put up, and new trenches dug, and big guns brought in on the railways, and saw a number of new French troops quartered in the dunes—all ominous signs of trouble to come.

The big military hospital at Beveren was well arranged—the barracks built around a large court and all connected, so that one did not have to go outside, as is generally the case. It stood on flat, unattractive land, but we were told that in summer the flower gardens were quite lovely. The doctors did not appear to be of quite as good a class as those with Dr. Depage, and the nurses seemed older and more tired, not as young or attractive as ours. But I was much impressed by the fine organisation and the cleanliness evident everywhere, in wards, operating-rooms, and disinfecting plant. Several *entrants* came into the receiving-room while we were there, one of them completely done for. The doctor who took us round said a good many wounded Germans had been brought in the past few days. He asked one of them how it seemed to be a prisoner, and the Boche answered, "I am glad."

On our way home we stopped at the farm which supplied the patients at Ocean Hospital with milk and vegetables. The sheep of the country were raised there, and cows that looked for all the world like our old red cattle at home, such as we used to pay forty or fifty dollars apiece for, but here they were worth at least a hundred and twenty-five. Dr. Depage was preserving here a special breed of horses, which had become almost extinct through the war because they were particularly good for artillery—small beasts but strong and sturdy, looking very much like Percheron colts.

Speaking of horses, those used in the Belgian Army looked well fed and handsome, and were mostly Irish. Even before the war, Irish horses were in general use for riding, though the big Percherons were employed for heavy work, of course.

One day I went to see the queen's school for frontier children. There were about five hundred youngsters there, all under seventeen, living in the usual wooden barracks. They had shower baths and hot water, and everything looked spick and span:—

> There is a spirit of youth and a sort of Kate-Greenaway look to it, with the curtains gathered back from the windows, and the shrubs and gay garden plots easing the right angles of the duck boards that run from door to door.

The pretty chapel had statues and relics from bombarded churches. Most of the teachers were nuns, except the superintendent and the man who taught gymnastics.

With a few exceptions, the children were not orphans; most of them had been sent back from homes nearer the front to be cared for here in comparative safety. The mother might come for them at any time if she were moving away from the front and could give them a home out of the danger zone. The fathers were of course in the army. The government would not allow even the orphans to be adopted by foreigners, for it wished them to remain Belgian subjects. As most of the children were from the immediate neighbourhood—Belgium Libre—they were nearly all Flemish.

One bright little chap about six years old had been brought in from the trenches, where he had lived for several months with the soldiers. He had been lost, and it was afterwards discovered that his parents had been killed. Another child had but one arm, the other having been destroyed by a bomb.

I went from one classroom to another, and the children sang and recited for me little songs and poems about their country or their lovely queen, whom they adored. They sang one American song, taught them by a Belgian nun who was, I am afraid, a little uncertain of her pronunciation. The children looked intelligent and well fed—I was surprised at the large amount of bread given each child. But then, the Belgians make most of their meal on bread and are more dependent on it than we are, often having two or three huge slices at each meal. The youngsters asked me for chocolates, and I was much distressed at not having thought to take some, but sent them candy later.

Those little blond children all seemed so innocent and sweet that I was very much touched. They were affectionate and confiding, much better mannered than our children of that age and class, and yet more dependent and less able to look out for themselves. When I came to say goodbye, several of them lifted their little faces to be kissed, and I should have been glad enough to bring them all home with me.

One morning in the operating-room I chanced to tell Her Majesty, who was working there, that I must be leaving Belgium in a few days, as my *permission* was nearly over. Not content with having done so much to make my stay there interesting, she arranged that I should have a day before leaving that I could never forget.

The *commandant* came with the motor and took me north along the sea. In the sand there were numberless holes, with soldiers popping in and out like gophers. I supposed of course that each hole led into an individual hut more or less like those round La Panne. But when we left the car and went down into one, I found to my astonishment that I was in a city under the sand, with continuous passageways to which the openings I had seen were merely occasional entrances.

We walked for miles through these underground tunnels, which were dark save where there was a spot of light from an entrance. The walls were made more or less solid by wood and sandbags, but I noticed that the side of the one bordering the sea was pitted with bullet holes. Opening off the criss-cross passages, which, though only two or three feet wide, served as the streets of this labyrinthine city, were alcoves, where the men had their sleeping-quarters.

Now and then, as we prowled along in single file, we met a soldier on duty, and passed big hidden searchlights and guns. It was such a maze that I marvelled how anyone could ever find his way about, even by the help of the signs which were stuck up here and there, much like those on motor roads.

Finally, branching off from the bullet-pocked alley, we came out into a cellar in Nieuport Bains. Still continuing on underground, only this time through cellar passages beneath the once famous bathing resort, it became so dark that we had to use the torchlight till we found a little lantern tucked in the wall and lighted that. At the end of these cellar passages was a room full of bottles and bandages, and echoing

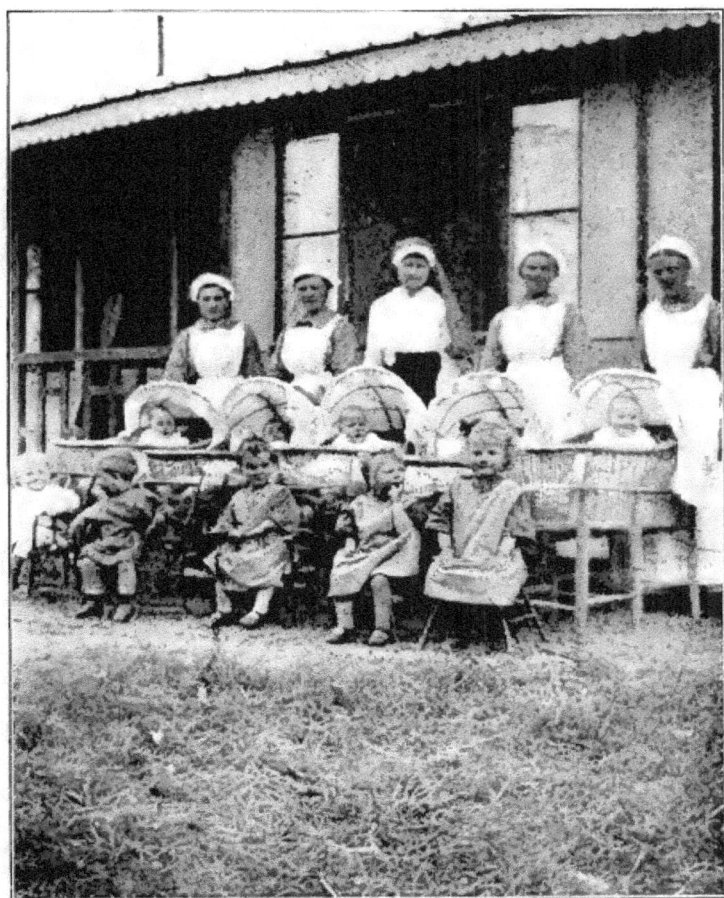

BABIES SAVED FROM THE FIRING-LINE

with shouts of laughter. There was no one there but ourselves, so the effect was uncanny till I looked through a hole in a wooden partition and saw some *brancardiers* playing cards.

Mounting some steps, we emerged for a moment into the daylight. Close by stood an ambulance, half-hidden by the wall of a demolished house. I was warned not to go out into the deserted street, as it was especially exposed. Some soldiers had been killed there only the day before. As it was, there was a constant loud crashing of guns, for we were very near the canal, on the other side of which were the Boches. Before the war, Nieuport Bains had been the prettiest and most fashionable of all the seashore resorts. Now there seemed little, if anything, left of the town. But, to tell the truth, I did not stay very long to see what it was like, for it did not seem a healthy place to linger, this spring of 1918.

Back again into the darkness, returning the little lantern to its place, we started to retrace our steps toward La Panne. Climbing up into the sunlight for a moment, we were crossing part of a sand dune above the buried city when a colonel in charge sent an orderly out to tell us to come in at once, as it was very dangerous there.

Our day did not end with our safe return to the motor, which was waiting where we had left it for this hazardous expedition. It came very near ending there, though, with just a prosaic ride back to La Panne, for the *commandant* was rather loath to take me to Nieuport itself. He said it was quite demolished and there had been a bad attack the day before. But on second thoughts, and after a little judicious persuasion, he changed his mind.

Nieuport is only two miles inland from the Bains, but the approach had two features that were new to me. The huts were made extraordinarily well, of mud and grass—I think they had been made by the British, but were occupied now by Belgians. Also, the branches of the trees along the road had been quite shot away, and their blackened stumps stuck up like broken fingers.

The ground was alive with soldiers under bumpy green mounds, and I must say they looked astonished at seeing me. The *commandant* said he thought no woman had ever been in that part before except the queen.

When it became too dangerous for the motor to go any farther, we got out and hid it behind the wall of a house—the only house left standing for miles about—and went the rest of the way on foot. Crossing a little bridge, we found ourselves in Nieuport, once the biggest town in the north of what is now Belgium Libre, but at present a mass of ruins.

From my *Spell of Belgium*, written several years ago, I take this paragraph about Nieuport, for it shows, I think, that judging from its past we need have no fear for the future of the plucky little city, desolate though it is today:—

> Nearer the mouth of the Yser was Nieuport, the "new port" made when the harbour across the river filled with sand during a terrific storm in the twelfth century . . . a quaint old town, with some really fine Gothic buildings, hidden by its sheltering mounds of sand from the hotels and villas of the beach, which is called Nieuport Bains to distinguish the resort from its moribund neighbour. Nieuport . . . was destroyed in 1388, after withstanding nine sieges. A hundred years later it was successfully defended against the French, the women and even the children fighting side by side with the men. It was destroyed again in the seventeen hundreds—three times, in fact. . . . A brave little town, among its grey-green sand dunes, with its ancient lighthouse and its empty, echoing square.

Returning to the place where we had left the motor, we climbed to the second storey of the house, which was half open and demolished, and had a good look out over the ruined city. Apparently, the house had been used for observation, for wooden steps remained, and small holes at the top through which one could see the flashes of the Boche guns, and the shells coming toward us across the canal and bursting a mile or so away.

Strewn along the road were scraps of ammunition and shrapnel, and I picked up a piece of an old cartridge to remember the place by, but I found a better souvenir than that—a horseshoe, which indeed brought me luck.

My *permission* was finished, but no word had come from Mrs. Daly, recalling me to work in France. This was not surprising, because, as I have said before, letters and telegrams were often delayed. I felt obliged to take matters into my own hands and return to Paris for orders.

The last night of my stay in La Panne arrived. I was feeling very sad, because they had all been so good to me, and I had had such unheard-of experiences for a woman. In the midst of my goodbyes, a servant came up and said the queen's lady-in-waiting was below and wished to see me. As I had already said goodbye to both her and her husband, and had sent messages to the king and the queen, I could not imagine why she had come.

To my complete surprise, she brought out a small box, a gift, she said, from Her Majesty. Opening it, I was delighted to find a decoration—the medal of Elisabeth. (See Appendix.)

Chapter 10

With Pershing's Boys

Then we'll tramp, tramp, tramp, and we'll fight, fight, fight,
For liberty and freedom, for justice, truth and right.
We'll fight on land or water, or high up in the air.
On mountains steep, in trenches deep, we'll fight, fight anywhere;
Till every nation, great or small, from despots shall be free
We'll fight to, make this wide, wide world safe for Democracy.

The first person I saw on getting back to Paris from La Panne was Dr. Lardenoir, my French *médecin-chef*. I asked him if the American nurses were working with him at the front again. The spring drive had begun, and the wounded were pouring in, so I was much surprised when he said that he was not ready for us. But Mrs. Daly, whom I went to see at once, said she was sure we would soon be needed, and urged me to remain in her unit until my return home in May. (See Appendix.)

The air raids were many and lively in Paris, and the mysterious long-range cannon, nicknamed "Bertha," was beginning to get in her work. The alarm was more terrifying than the raids themselves. Fire engines went whistling, wailing, shrieking through the streets, frightening the inhabitants. As the German flyers usually came late in the evening, when the alarm sounded the dark corridors of the hotel would swarm with strangely clad people—women in wrappers, with their hair flying, and funny fat men in striped pyjamas.

There was a full moon the week of my stay in Paris, so we had a raid almost every night. I went to the theatre three times, but each time the signal came before the play was over, and the curtain was dropped. There was never any panic in the audience. People calmly got up and sauntered out of the theatre, while the band continued to play as if nothing were happening. We would make our way home as best we could, in the dark. I always managed to have a little supper waiting in my sitting-room at the hotel, and we would sit there enjoying ourselves while the raid went on.

"Bertha" began her activities about daybreak, and between my friends who stayed late o' nights, and my enemies the Boches who came early in the morning, I didn't have very much chance to sleep. Sometimes we would go down and look out of the front door, to see the French aviators, with their lights, flying about over the city. Now and then you would hear a bomb drop, but it was always hard to tell where it landed. The first few days of the long range gun-fire the shops in Paris were closed, but after that, everybody went about as usual.

My room was on the top floor, which is supposed to be the most dangerous, and I was told that it was better to go downstairs, not only when the raids were on, but when the big gun began her day's work. But it is especially annoying, if you are very tired and sleepy, to have to wake up at five in the morning and go down to the ground floor. For three days I did it with the others, but after that stayed in bed and had my coffee there. Afterwards the Ritz was struck by a bomb, and this room of mine quite demolished.

Only once during my entire time in Paris did I go into a cellar, and that was chiefly out of curiosity. At the hotel where a friend of mine was staying, there was supposed to be a particularly safe *cave*, and one night after the theatre I went down to see what it was like. It was disappointing, for it was just like any cellar, only with people sitting about playing cards by the light of candles.

Palm Sunday, on the way to Notre Dame, some of us walked across the Tuileries Gardens almost in a direct line from the Place Vendôme and saw a big hole made the night before by "Bertha." I couldn't help thinking of a great hen making a nest to lay an egg. While we stood there looking at it, there was a whiz and a whine and a frightful explosion, and "Bertha" had dropped another *obus*.

Crossing the river, we continued on to the cathedral to say our prayers. It was a warm, sunny day, and after the service we went out into the Bois and had luncheon under the trees in a restaurant garden where the birds were singing, and afterwards hired a boat and rowed about on what at home would be called a frog pond.

I was beginning to get rather tired of Paris when a long-wished-for chance arrived to see something of the American front. One night,

Countess Castre, who was dining with me, suggested that I make her a little visit at her *château*, which was near General Pershing's headquarters. Mrs. Daly granted me permission to go for a few days, and the Red Cross gave me a pass. So, as in the fairy tale, my wishes came true, and I started off for Lorraine with the countess from the Gare de l'Est on a Thursday night at eight o'clock.

I mention the exact time because at that very same hour the next evening a bomb was dropped on the Gare de l'Est. It was on that day, too—Good Friday—that the Church of Saint Gervais in Paris was shelled and so many people were killed.

The countess and I had to sit up all night. At three in the morning we stopped for a few minutes at Troyes. The station was filled with refugees from Châlons-sur-Marne, some of them so pathetic that I opened my suit case and shared my warm clothing with them.

It was still early morning when we arrived at our destination, a pretty little town named Bar-sur-Aube, surrounded by low hills. Through this wooded country we motored on to the beautiful *château* of Cirey, which stands in a park, and is famous for the things that happened there in days long past. Once upon a time it furnished a hiding-place for the great Cardinal Richelieu, and for nine years it was the home of Voltaire.

At that time the *château* was the property of the Marquis du Châtelet, a noble "of ancient house and dilapidated fortune," and Voltaire was the guest of his wife. Madame du Chatelet was not beautiful, but she was a student and evidently a woman of considerable ability. When she died, the countess told me, Voltaire and the marquis agreed that they would open together the locket which she had always worn, the contents of which neither of them had ever seen. Each of them hoped it might be his own picture and feared that it might be the other's, but to their surprise they found the portrait of a third man!

It poured so hard all day that I did not see the park to advantage, though I wandered about through the lovely lanes and among the farm buildings in spite of the rain. One of the houses on the estate was being made ready for some American officers. The countess was very good to my countrymen, and from time to time had her *château* filled with them. The picturesque village nearby was crowded with our soldiers. At the post office the post mistress assured me that the American troops behaved very well and that they liked to have them there. Someone else told me that they had stolen most of the countess's chickens!

That evening some American officers came to dinner. I can never forget the date, which was the 29th of March, for on that day Pershing gave his splendid message to the Allies, which I read in the papers there:—

> I come to say to you that the American people would hold it a great honour for our troops were they engaged in the present battle. I ask it of you in my name and in that of the American people. There is at this moment no other question than that of fighting. Infantry, artillery, aviation—all that we have are yours, to dispose of as you will. Others are coming that will be as numerous as necessary. I have come to say to you that the American people would be proud to be engaged in the greatest battle in history.

That speech made us very happy, it expressed so vigorously just what all of us were feeling, and what we knew the people at home were feeling, too—we wanted to get into the fight for which we had been preparing.

Years before, when my husband and I were out in the Philippines with our Secretary of War, we had seen a good deal of General Pershing, who was then stationed at Zamboanga, on one of the southern islands. So, when the Count de Chambrun, who had married a cousin of ours, came over next morning and suggested taking me to headquarters to call on the commander-in-chief, I fairly jumped at the chance. The count is a descendant of Lafayette, and was liaison officer on Pershing's staff.

We set off in the motor over the winding roads, passing a Roman tower—for Lorraine holds much ancient history—and crossing a river at the foot of the valley, where a soldier was on guard. Mounting a steep slope where a ruined castle stood on a cliff overhanging the valley, we came at last to the top of the hill and the town of Chaumont. In this old French town, it seemed incongruous to see the peaked hats of the New World. It made me feel quite homesick.

It is an interesting coincidence that our troops should be stationed at Chaumont, for it was there that the earlier allies, in 1814, signed a solemn covenant not to lay down their arms until they had overthrown their common enemy—in that case, Napoleon Bonaparte.

General Pershing's headquarters consisted of a large, handsome building with a huge courtyard in front. After waiting for a few moments in an outer room where there were a number of army officers

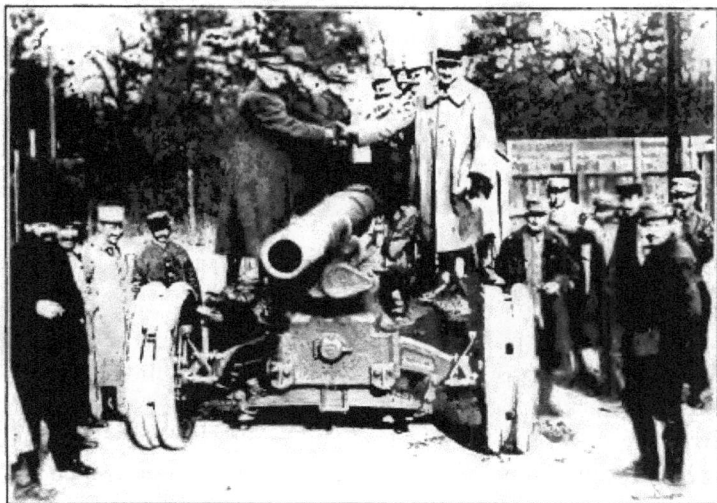

AMERICANS CONGRATULATING THEIR FRENCH COMRADES
ON THE COMPLETION OF THE FIRST 155-MM. GUN
BUILT BY THE FRENCH GOVERNMENT FOR
THE UNITED STATES ARMY

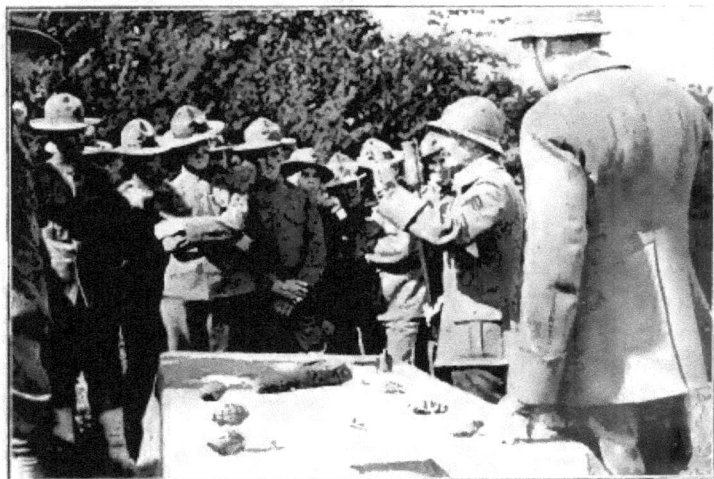

A LESSON ON HAND GRENADES

busy at desks, we were shown into the private office of the commander-in-chief.

He was looking extremely well, and we chatted about the old days in the Philippines rather than about present-day matters. As I was leaving, he asked me to dine with him on my return through Chaumont a few days later.

I had a jolly luncheon that day at a lovely little villa in which lived six American officers, all old friends of ours. One of them. Colonel M., decided that he would put on a new uniform, for he was just starting for Italy with our American Secretary of War. So, I fastened the leaves on his shoulder straps and sewed on the many-colored ribbons which showed his service.

From Chaumont we motored on to General Edwards's headquarters, which were then in a beautiful French *château* on a wooded hillside. One of the windows overlooked a little valley where, by the river, I could see our khaki-coloured tents and the familiar American mule. There were only a few tents, though, for most of our soldiers were billeted, after the French method, in the little towns round about.

As it was still raining, General Edwards insisted that I should spend the night there rather than try to go on in the motor after dark. Besides, he wanted me to see the Massachusetts commissioners, friends of ours, who were dining there.

It was here I heard the story of how, when a German plane was brought down a short time before, some American soldiers, thinking that the pilot might have torn up some papers and thrown them away, hunted this part of the country over. Sure enough, they found the bits of a map, which, when put together, disclosed some very important information, shall we say? about submarine bases.

The army men certainly were good. Next morning, they sent me on to Neufchâteau and deposited me at a canteen kept by two Red Cross women. One of them, General Scott's daughter, was presiding over a small counter in a green tent by a railway station. Just outside was an army kitchen where an American soldier was making coffee. Troops, both French and American, were constantly passing through. In the town were Red Cross storehouses guarded by several men who, with the aid of their motors, kept the many dispensaries provided with supplies, as well as several large hospitals for the civilian population.

Before the war there were no doctors, even, in this part of the country, and such institutions as those I saw were really very much needed, not only for persons injured by bombs, but for those who were ill in the community. It is said that there is a long chain of Red Cross dispensaries stretching from the northern part of the frontier away down to the Mediterranean.

Of a different sort was the military hospital No. 18, which was eventually to consist of seven thousand beds. At this time there were only a thousand, and they were building slowly—very slowly, for lumber was difficult to get. Since seeing this hospital, I have heard of others that are to be even larger.

The location was ideal, a lovely little valley. I went about from barrack to barrack, talking with the soldiers. A great many of them had been gassed. When I inquired if any of them would like to send messages home, quite a number gave me their names and addresses and asked me to tell their friends that they were getting on all right, and were well taken care of—even the worst cases wished their people told that they would soon be well. There was no complaining of any kind, and a splendid spirit existed. They did say that their letters had not seemed to reach home, and that they received very few, but I am glad to learn that since then the mail service has been improved. (See Appendix.)

Everything I saw or heard while in France leads me to feel that I can vouch for the statement made by a man who has investigated conditions more thoroughly than most:

> I may sum up in a sentence, the weeks of investigation in France, and uncounted interviews with all the men I could meet who are supposed to have special knowledge on the subject, by saying that the young men of the American Expeditionary Force are better, morally and physically, than were these same young men at home, or than are an equal number of their fellows at home.

There was a big Y.M.C.A. building in Neufchâteau, and their coffee, reading-room, and movies seemed to be greatly appreciated. In fact, the American soldier at that time was most enthusiastic about the "Y," which seems to be exceptionally well organised. The only criticism I heard was that the huts were going up slowly—due to the lack of lumber—and that the Association charged well for the food provided. (See Appendix.)

A worker in one of their canteens wrote me not long ago:

> I am with a regiment that comes from within thirty miles of my own home. I love them. Irish-Americans with blue eyes put in with a smutty finger, and—such language! I should think an

old-fashioned Y.M.C.A. worker would curl up and die!

That night I spent with Miss Scott at Neufchâteau, going on next day to Toul. Our road led past Domremy, the small hamlet where Joan was born, with low white houses, lining its one street, which ends at the church. It was on a hill, only a short distance away, that the Maid heard her "Voices."

I had seen the French and English Armies on the move, and now had the good fortune to see Uncle Sam's boys on their way to the front-line trenches. It was pouring rain, and quite cold, but the men looked healthy and cheerful in spite of the weather. Even the horses looked fat and well cared for.

For miles the straight road was covered with army wagons, motors, guns and loads of ammunition. Besides the big guns there were little ones mounted on two wheels which I had not seen before, each drawn by a mule. With the driver in his campaign hat the outfit looked distinctly American. But the peaked hat is fast disappearing for the more appropriate fatigue cap; with this change the "Yanks" are losing their identity, as the caps are much like those of other armies. It was always a surprise to me not to find regiments marching at the front, but as a matter of fact they never travel on foot in large numbers. There are often soldiers straggling along among the guns, but most of them are transported either by motors or trains.

I was proud to hear—what of course I knew must be true—that our boys are fearless fighters, and that the French consider them much like the Canadians.

At Toul, one of the oldest towns in Lorraine—it has been the seat of a bishop for a dozen centuries—I was deposited at Dr. Ladd's Red Cross hospital for frontier women and children. It occupied old brick barracks on the top of a hill, and the doctors whom I talked with seemed more concerned with the destruction of bugs and cooties than anything else. The children all had their hair cut short and were kept very clean. Miss Bradley, who was working there, has given a lively description of the patients in a letter from which I am going to quote:

A procession is passing my window, probably the drollest I have ever seen. The refugee women, armed with a clean towel apiece, are on their way to the bath house for probably the very first bath in their lives. Grandma, with her bent back and white hair; middle-aged, frowsy women, who have never had time in their hard-worked lives to think of a bath—and *mon Dieu!* they show it—young nursing mothers of twenty or so who still retain a fleeting resemblance to their once comely girlhood—all must pass today through their ordeal, under pain of expulsion from the *asile*.

To quote from another source:

> From Noyon came a peasant woman, leaving the farm that she worked at night because the German shells kept her down in her cellar during the day—on a ten-day vacation to give birth to her sixth child. She stayed two weeks, and then left, straining the child to her breast for one last hug before she said goodbye to her baby and returned to her farm. 'I have a good crop,' she said simply, as she put down her child, 'France needs me more than I need my baby.'

Dr. Ladd's wife was doing a wonderful work at her studio in Paris. She was a well-known sculptress, but had given that up for the moment and was making masks to cover disfigured faces. She used a photograph of the soldier which showed how he looked before he was wounded, and made a mask of copper or silver to resemble it and cover the part of the face which was seared or gone. The mask was made as light as possible, and was held on with bows behind the ears, like spectacles. In some cases, just a nose was put on, so well that it was hardly noticeable, sometimes a chin, or half a face. As a rule, the patients cannot eat or sleep in their masks, but of course can see and breathe through them, and as they are painted in very lifelike flesh tints, their wearers can go into the streets and theatres without feeling that people are shrinking from them.

Dr. Ladd took me to Sebastopol, the hospital nearest the trenches for our "Sammies." I was glad to find there some of our very best surgeons. Major Gosman, an old friend of ours, was in charge; we found him in a little portable house, greatly rushed with his work.

Many things here attracted my attention, but I was especially interested in a laundry on wheels, run by a motor—something that I had never seen before, though it was made in France. It was working out of doors and was in use day and night—a most necessary and convenient thing for temporary hospitals.

A Ford was to take me back to the American headquarters at Chaumont, where I was to dine with General Pershing that evening. What a trip I had in the rain! For a while the machine ran very well, and we flew through little villages where Yanks were singing "Yankee Doodle" and other old-time American songs. Then a tire blew out, just as it was getting dark, and we had to stop to change it. While waiting for that, I had a bit of a chat with one of our men who was cleaning his boots at a pump. He was from New England, too, and we exchanged good wishes for each other's safe return to the old Bay State, and he waved me a cheery goodbye as the Ford once more whizzed off into the darkness.

We did not whiz very long, though, for "Henry" got tired and absolutely refused to climb the hill at Neufchâteau. As he did not respond to treatment, it was decided that I had better try another machine. So, a second Ford was obtained, with a very small boy to drive it, and I set off once more with high hopes.

In spite of the blackness of the night and the pouring rain we went at a terrific speed, for the child had been impressed with the necessity of getting me to Chaumont in time for dinner, whatever happened. Slipping, sliding, skidding, uphill and down—why we were not killed I do not know. As it was, the general had finished dinner when I got there, but he very kindly took me in and gave me a most welcome bite, and sat with me while I ate it. I was too cold and shaken to pieces by Henry to talk very intelligently, and the only thing which I remember General Pershing's saying was that he was very much troubled by the lack of ships.

Count de Chambrun came for me and said it would be much better for me to sleep at their villa than to go to the hotel, that I could have Colonel M.'s room, for he had gone to Italy. He promised to take me to the train next morning at five o'clock, and I was indeed grateful for being personally conducted.

The trip back to Paris was rather interesting, although the train was delayed. The drive was on and the troop trains of course went first. There were motors on some of the freight cars, and huge 155 guns painted with great blotches of green and brown. From the windows of the passenger coaches hung men in horizon-blue caps and coats.

The time passed quickly because I was amused by a French girl in the compartment giving lessons to two doughboys. The last sentence I heard before dropping off to sleep was something about a "camouflaged baby doll."

Chapter 11

Working in the Drive

I am sorry I cannot tell you where I am because I am not allowed to say. But I venture to state that I am not where I was,
but where I was before I left here to go to where I have just
come from. (*Punch.*)

When I got back to Paris from the American front, I found a message waiting for me at the hotel. It ordered me to be ready to leave
next morning with another nurse for the French front, but it made
no mention of the place where we were to be stationed. Red Cross
workers are supposed to have as little interest in geography as soldiers.

The suit cases with my uniforms were to be packed and sent to
the nurse's hotel that night, so that all might be forwarded together. I
knew it would be necessary to take a good supply of clothes, for we
might be away several weeks, and although washing is only done once
in a thousand years at the front, nurses must always look spick and
span. As it was still very cold, plenty of woollen things had to be taken,
and blankets and pillows besides. Of course, as usually happened, I
couldn't begin to close my bags and had to have the whole hotel force
up to stand on them. To my dismay, it was dinner time before I was
half through my arrangements, and guests were coming—an American general, a Belgian officer, and a French countess.

It was only after they had gone that it occurred to me that I had
better call up the nurse and decide upon our meeting the next morning. I supposed of course that she had my pass. But imagine my horror
when I was told she did not have it, and had not seen it, and did not
know anything about it. As it was too late to do anything in regard to
it then, my companion advised me to meet her just the same. She had
her pass and was going by train, but said I could go without papers on

the motor which was to take hospital materials all the way to Compiègne. From there we were to continue on to an evacuated hospital. She was very mysterious as to just where we were going. Mrs. Daly, it appeared, had already gone to the front with a few of her nurses to join our *médecin-chef*, Dr. Lardenoir.

Well, I finished packing my trunk, which was to be left in the storeroom of the hotel, and made up six boxes for my *poilus* as well, writing a letter for each box. Thinking I might never get a hot bath again, I took two, one at midnight, the other at three in the morning. There was time for a little sleep, and then I got up, at five, and went to meet my companion at her hotel.

Another blow! Just as I was getting into the Red Cross motor for Compiègne, as I supposed, the driver calmly informed me that he didn't have a permit to take us out of Paris! He would be obliged to send the hospital supplies by rail. The Red Cross headquarters did not open till nine o'clock, and the train for Compiègne started in fifteen minutes. I had visions of being left on the sidewalk and perhaps waiting for ten days to get my pass, but the nurse said that it would do no harm for me to try and go by train, if possible. The only thing to do was to go to the station.

I shall never forget that morning. The luggage was heaped high in the motor, and when the driver and the nurse were settled there was no place for another human being to sit. But I was determined not to be left behind at the start, so I scrambled up onto the machine and perched myself on top of the pyramid of bags, hanging on for dear life, with cape flapping and veil flying, as we rattled off through the streets of Paris.

When we reached the depot, my heart was in my mouth as I marched bravely up to the ticket office. In my hand I held the best I had to offer—my red identification card! There was a crowd around the window, the man was very busy. He saw that I wore a nurse's uniform, and that was enough—without a word he handed me a ticket. Seizing it joyfully, I jumped aboard the train for Compiègne and began to wonder what would happen next.

Those were strange and thrilling days, when millions of Germans were rushing down upon us, pushing our armies before them. Refugees were piling into Paris from Noyon and Compiègne. The whole city was astir with movement and unrest, a very different Paris from any that I had ever known.

People were running to the banks and drawing out their money.

As we thought the Germans might really enter Paris, I had cabled to my husband to see if I could take out his money as well as my own, thinking to save it and transfer it to London. He did not realise the situation in the least, but thought I needed funds, and not only wired me to draw on his account, but cabled me still more money. During the delay the banks decided not to allow a soul to transfer deposits to London, so ours were left to their fate.

Notwithstanding the excitement in Paris, it was much more exciting at the real front, for the spring drive had become alarming. Battles had been raging for days. Our *auto-chir* at Cugny, which the British had taken over, had been destroyed; four of the doctors had been shot by the Germans. The British Army had been retreating—eighty thousand of their men dead or prisoners.

> The bombardment which opened at 5.30 a.m. on March 21st on the whole front was extremely heavy. On a large part of the front the Germans had an average of one gun to every twelve or fifteen yards, besides a great number of trench mortars, which they used to cut wire and pound our forward positions. The bombardment of the front lines was probably as heavy as has been seen in this war. . . . It was probably the greatest artillery concentration ever known.

As another newspaper put it:—

> The days of 1914 seem to have returned. The impression is as if the era of the migration of peoples had been revived. Streams of men, animals, wagons and war munitions of all kinds rolled forward. From a high viewpoint one sees them winding like endless giant snakes over the valleys and hills.

All the dressing-stations behind the trenches had to be evacuated the first day. The regular method of evacuating hospitals was this: first, the nurses were sent ahead in an ambulance lorry; then every patient who could walk had to take the road on foot; the severely wounded were loaded into ambulances and sent off. The hospital staff, left behind, set to work to destroy whatever there was no chance of taking. The surgical instruments were put into handcarts, and the doctors themselves in many cases pushed them along the road, mile after mile, in the darkness. Several wheeled their precious loads even forty miles before coming to a place of safety.

Some of the officers were so worn out with their ceaseless care of the wounded and their marching that they swayed about like drunken men.

When we reached the station at Compiègne, I was confronted by a man who demanded passes. I waved my red card at him and hurried through the gate with the other nurse. There was a jam of people, and he let me go.

We walked to the hotel, through the empty streets of the beautiful old town. It was absolutely deserted, with freshly made *obus* holes in the cobblestones and walls. In the past it was the home of Marie Antoinette and of the later kings of France at one time or another during their reigns, and the favourite residence of Napoleon III.

Fortunately, the superb *façade* of the *château* had not been damaged at all, though the hotel opposite had been struck several times and abandoned. Over its door we noticed a red cross, and inside discovered Mrs. Daly and our nurses, who had taken possession and had been sleeping in the cellar. They said that every evening the town was heavily bombed.

They had opened a canteen and dispensary, and for the moment the nurses became waitresses as well, while some Red Cross men handed out cigarettes to the passing soldiers and chocolate to the refugees. There were two or three families who were too old or too ill to leave the town, and these we also took under our wing.

When the inhabitants fled from Compiègne they left their cats and dogs prowling about the streets or locked in their houses. There was no food for them, so they were collected and killed. At the hotel I heard the crying of a dog, and after some searching discovered the little beast, a mangy old fox terrier who had evidently been forgotten. All I had to give him was a lump of sugar and some water, but the poor little thing was very grateful and wanted to stay with me. I was obliged, of course, to turn him over to a Red Cross man, and heard that he went to the dogs' paradise the next day.

We were sent to Royalieu, a hospital four miles north of Compiègne. It had been evacuated a week before, and required considerable cleaning and putting in order before it could be again used. (Since I left it has been evacuated again.) While cleaning it, the nurses came into the hotel for their meals. At noon and night, we jumped into a huge *camion*, huddled in with the French servants, our gas masks hanging about our necks. It was so crowded that at every corner I expected the machine would upset, but it was so well driven by one of the women of the unit that there were no accidents. As I look back upon those first hectic days, the trips to Compiègne for meals stand out as particularly amusing and exciting. The meals themselves were not so amusing, for the cook, a returned refugee, was drunk most of the time, and one night poured kerosene on the meat.

More nurses joined us, French and English, and it did not take us long to get things ready at Royalieu, although conditions there were extremely primitive and it was at best far from comfortable. There were absolutely no sanitary arrangements, and what water we had did not look inviting.

One of the most distressing things to me was the lack of liquid to drink, for we were too busy to boil the water, and even though I had been inoculated for typhoid and para-typhoid I did not like to drink it without taking that precaution. Sometimes late at night we made coffee, but I was driven to drinking up my whole bottle of Pond's Extract before I got through.

The hospital stood on low land by a canal, a huge establishment of forty barracks or more, built of brick, with streets running between them.

Mounting stone steps to the centre of the main building, one entered a long corridor from which opened several morgue-like *salles* of stone. These were reserved for our sleeping-quarters and for storing our supplies. The other barracks, quite like ours, were for the wounded.

The first thing to do was to clean our sleeping-quarters from top to bottom; stone floors and walls and the one big window at the end, all had to be scoured and scrubbed, for they were not only dirty, but nobody knew whether infectious cases hadn't been cared for there before.

Eight American nurses slept in one room, the British nurses in another, the French in a third. After cleaning everything, we lugged in our cots and mattresses and made our beds. Each of us had a small tin table, and there was a shelf all around the room for our things. Fortunately, the space near the window fell to me, so I had a little light and air, but on the other hand, it was conspicuous, as soldiers were constantly passing and looking in, until we put up blankets for curtains.

As soon as our own quarters were settled, we began opening up one barrack after another for the wounded. We dragged in iron bedsteads and mattresses and sorted out blankets and sheets. I was nick-named "Handy Andy of the Mattress Brigade." There were about fourteen beds in each *salle* for the soldiers, and six *salles* in each barrack, besides a linen room and a small one—*pansement salle*—at each end, where wounds were dressed. One ward was kept for the officers, but it was no different from the others except that it had ten beds instead of fourteen and they were larger and more comfortable. We tried to find linen that had not been stained, and covered the beds with pretty chintzes.

There were several *infirmières* and orderlies on duty in each building and a nurse in each *pansement salle*. The operating was all done in a big green caterpillar tent that had been set up outside. As we were an *auto-chir* hospital, we were used only for the very seriously wounded, and our *équipe* was given only surgical work, as at Cugny. Just as soon as we were ready to receive the soldiers, they began to come in from the trenches. They were terribly shot to pieces, and many had head wounds, which were perhaps the worst of all. But even when the *poilus* were suffering tortures, they never forgot to say some pleasant words.

During my first days in the ward I became interested in a blond man who had been shot in the head. As he did not speak for a long time after he was brought in, I thought perhaps he was a German. However, to be on the safe side, I asked him if he were English.

"No, French," he said, adding, "and are you American?"

When I answered that I was, he said, very sweetly, "*Très gentil!*"

Afterwards I was transferred to the *pansement salle* and lost track of him for a while. Later he was brought in, very much worse, but I never heard whether he pulled through or not.

Another man in my ward had both legs and an arm broken. Out of eight brought into the *triage*, five died in one night. It is terribly hard—you want to do so much for them, and yet there is often so little that you can do, just make them clean and a little more comfortable, and warm with hot drinks and water bottles.

One day a hundred wounded poured into the *triage*. (See Appendix.) Among them were a German officer and a private. The officer was quite badly injured, the soldier had only a slight wound in one hand, so we decided it would be pleasanter for all concerned if the private waited on the officer. But several days later, to our great amazement, while lying quietly on his bed, the private died, and no one could find out how it happened. I never heard that the mystery was ever cleared up.

The kitchen had at last been started at the hospital, presided over by a lop-sided old woman and a sixteen-year-old boy, so we no longer were obliged to go to the hotel in town for our meals.

A few refugees had begun to return to Compiègne, and we noticed that one or two shops had been reopened. In the evening you would see the inhabitants crossing the square with their mattresses and all their valuables, to spend the night in the hotel cellar.

There was no cellar at Royalieu to flee to when the Boche flying machines dropped bombs, but we felt safe enough, thinking that the Germans did not purposely bomb hospitals, unless troops were quartered nearby or there were bridges or manufacturing plants in the vicinity which they wished to destroy. In fact, we felt quite as safe as in Paris, where the aeroplane raids and the big gun "Bertha" kept us awake night after night.

One bomb did drop within half a mile, and eleven came down early one morning within a couple of miles of us, but this was because the Boches were trying to destroy the railway bridge at Compiègne. From my window at the hospital I counted seven balloons hovering over the trenches, and saw airplanes constantly passing. I learned to recognise the difference in sound between the aircraft. The French had a steadier "*burr*" and the Germans more of a "*tuff-tuff.*"

My time was up. Moreover, I had a bad cold, and was nearly exhausted. So, I was to leave Royalieu, and Mrs. Daly, and the staff, and return to America. Everybody was so kind that I was sorry to leave— even the *médecin-chef* wrote something nice in my *livret*, or hospital book.

Some of the others when they left had given little presents to the head surgeon. So, on my last day, seeing, as I thought in my hurry, a group of doctors together in the street, I believed it a good moment to say goodbye and thank them for their kindness, at the same time offering my little gift to the *médecin-chef*. But when it was all over, the nurses who were with me declared that I had said my *adieus* not only to the doctors but to two generals! They thought it a great joke. "The *médecin-chef* looked so embarrassed, poor man! The generals must have thought you were leaving in a rage and returning him his presents." But I'm not sure even now that they weren't really doctors.

I started off from Royalieu in a *camion*, sitting inside on a bag of soiled clothes with an empty oil can at my back.

On the way several passengers were picked up, one of them a man whom I had known in Boston years ago. He had been sent up here with a motor kitchen which had broken down on the way, and seeing our *camion* had begged a ride to Paris.

133

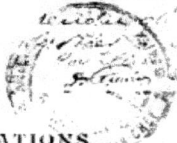

AFFECTATIONS

DATES	FORMATIONS	GRADES	OBSERVATIONS
[illegible] 191[illegible]	[illegible]	Infirmière	Madame Anderson infirmière [illegible] [illegible] de zèle et de [illegible] dévouement. Collaboratrice intelligente et attentive des chirurgiens [illegible]

AFFECTATIONS

DATES	FORMATIONS	GRADES	OBSERVATIONS

As we went through Compiègne many troops were passing, and Red Cross men were stationed at the street corners giving them cigarettes. The army horses looked thin in spite of their shaggy coats, the *poilus* in their faded uniforms seemed cold and tired.

I had to have several passes in order to leave France for England, consequently we stopped at a town somewhat aside from the usual route to Paris to get the first one. Mrs. Daly telephoned the day before to have the permit ready, but of course when I got there it was not signed, and the officer who should have put his name to it was not to be found. No one in the office knew where he was nor when he would be back. It was not until we announced our intention of waiting there till the officer returned, if it took all day, that someone suddenly remembered where he was and sent for him. We went out for a bite of luncheon, and on our return the papers had been signed and stamped.

Along the way we met endless troops and guns and *camions*, all on the road to the trenches. Several towns through which we passed had been partly destroyed, the bombing being always especially heavy round the railway stations and bridges. Some of this damage had been done in 1914, but much of it during the last drive.

A funny lot we must have looked as we entered the crowded streets of Paris, covered with dust, and descended with our battered bags and soiled wash at the fashionable hotel in the Place Vendôme.

CHAPTER 12

No Man's Children

Each time I returned to Paris I found conditions changed. The hotel was now almost deserted, for it stood on the edge of "Bertha's" path. The big gun was trained on the Gare de l'Est, the Tuileries, and the stations and government buildings on the other side of the river.

The food restrictions had also become more severe. Bread tickets were necessary at the hotel, and the tea-places had all been closed. Only tea and lemon could be procured in your own rooms. No cakes could be bought, and it was almost impossible to get crackers. Of course, no butter was served. Nevertheless, there were little things, such as fruit, honey, dates, and jam, which the hotel provided. You could find enough to eat, in one way or another, and could even ask a friend to tea.

Having a few days on my hands before leaving France, I used the time to see something of the work which the American Red Cross was doing for twenty thousand fatherless children who had come under its care. All of them were dirty and many of them ill and maimed from bombs when they were gathered together and distributed among the various colonies established for them, in different parts of France and Belgium. Each home was under the direction of doctors and nurses, and the little waifs were instructed by teachers and nuns. Mrs. Bliss, wife of the secretary of the American Embassy, was one of the moving spirits in this work, and certainly deserves a great deal of credit.

One of these institutions was located at Dandier, a monastery in the centre of France. The American Red Cross Commissioner for Belgium was good enough to take me to see the five hundred children sheltered there. They had been shipped out of Liége through Switzerland by the Germans, all by themselves, with no one to look after them.

How these little people made their journey to their new home has been touchingly described in a Red Cross bulletin:—

Five hundred children, travel-worn after three days in a closed train coming from Belgian provinces, crossed the frontier last night and reached Évian at dawn. Although so young that they did not know their own ages, they had travelled all that time motherless and unaccompanied. When the train stopped, they poured out into the streets, shaking hands with every bystander and crying, "*Vive la France!*" and "*Vive la Belgique!*"
Trumpeters, after the fashion of the Pied Piper of Hamelin, led the dancing, shouting throng to the casino—all except a few sick children who were carried in Red Cross ambulances. At the casino they all received food, flags were distributed, and songs were sung. Even very small children knew the words of the "*Brabançonne*" and the "*Marseillaise*," but some of them were so tired that they slept right through the music. (See Apendix.)

Our long trip from Paris was full of interest. It was a day's journey southward, through the famous *château* district. At Chartres I had a glimpse of the massive cathedral with its superb western towers. It is a common saying in France that "the towers of Chartres, the nave of Amiens, the choir of Beauvais, and the portal of Rheims would together make a perfect cathedral." Passing a big aviation camp and Orleans, the scene of the Maid's great triumph, we left the train at the station of Pompadour.

A huge *camion* was waiting for us—much to our relief, for we had half expected to walk the eight miles to the monastery. In the truck were a chauffeur and a German prisoner, who took charge of our luggage. There was a rifle in the car, put there to use in case the Boche tried to escape. The chauffeur said he didn't think there was much chance of that, though, for the prisoner seemed quite contented and did his work well. After the flat, devastated part of the north, so many times overrun by armies, it was a treat to see the beautiful hilly country, covered with trees.

The grounds of the great Carthusian monastery were surrounded by a heavy stone wall, above which the towers of chapels appeared. Between two rows of fine trees a *vista* was seen of the huge entrance gate and the courtyard beyond. Inside, in addition to the usual massive buildings, were twenty small houses inhabited not long ago by silent, white-cowled monks. On the ground floor of each were two rooms—

a woodshed and a workshop. Steps led up to a room above, part of which was used as a study, the rest as dormitory, oratory, and refectory in one. Attached to each house was a tiny garden, where the Carthusian found his only recreation. Through a little sliding shutter beside the door the brothers received their coarse and simple food. Only once a week was their solitude ever broken—on Sundays their white cowls could be seen outside the grounds. St, Bruno, the founder of the Carthusians, bound his followers by the severest rules, which they have observed so faithfully that the order has never needed to be reorganised.

What a contrast within those grim, damp walls today! The little houses have become classrooms, and the courtyards are filled with noisy, romping children.

As it was growing dark when we arrived, we saw but little of the institution that night. Supper—a meagre meal—was given us in the long, bare refectory. It was followed by coffee in the matron's room, reached through an endless corridor where a row of sleeping tots lay tucked into their beds.

I, too, went to bed early. My room was big, empty and cold. I simply crept between the blankets without undressing, so it was not difficult to get up at an early hour to attend mass in the chapel. This had only a dirt floor and a few rough wooden benches, where many children were praying. The priest asked the commissioner for a little money to finish the chapel, and I was able to get a few chairs and things to make the nurses a bit more comfortable. I was glad to do this, for I far preferred my own work at the front with wounded soldiers in barracks to the damp stone walls of the monastery and the constant battle to keep off children's diseases.

In spite of several cases of measles and diphtheria at this time, the five hundred children on the whole looked healthy, and their clothes were neat and clean. Their food was simple but plentiful. The nurses, teachers, and doctors, both American and Belgian, seemed to take a real pride in making the place a model establishment for the little wanderers from the invaded country, waifs from No Man's Land.

In the morning the children were gathered in the great courtyard, the boys going through physical exercises, the girls singing at their games. Later, we saw them in the classrooms, where they proved intelligent and eager to answer the questions put to them by the Red Cross commissioner.

In the afternoon, several hundred pupils marched into a hall and sang to us in Flemish, French, and English—they seemed to love do-

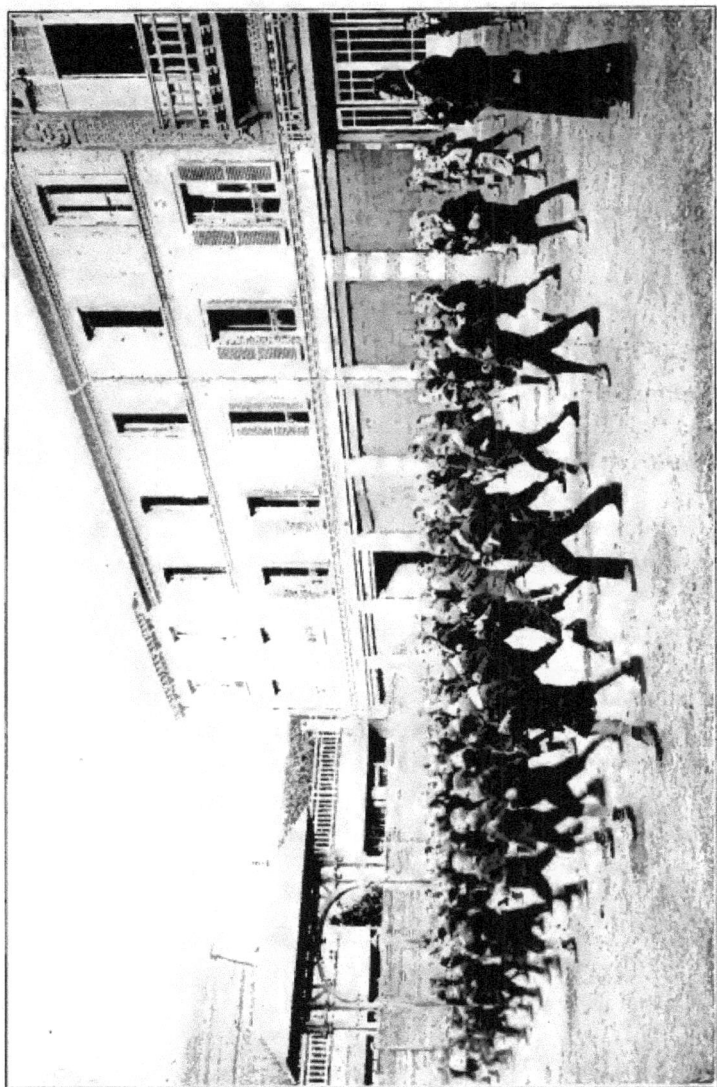

GYMNASTIC DRILL OF BELGIAN CHILDREN

ing it, even if they did sing out of tune.

After a pleasant walk over the hills near the monastery, we motored back to the town of Pompadour, in time to have a glimpse of the *château* given by Louis XV to his mistress, Madame de Pompadour. What a strange story it is! At nine years of age, singled out by a fortune-teller as the future mistress of the king, from that time on she was educated with that sole end in view. Like Napoleon, she believed in her star. To conquer the king was her aim, and to do this, she pursued him. When he went to the hunt in the forest of Sénart, she passed him again and again.

> In the midst of the escort, of the horses and dogs, sometimes dressed in blue and seated in a rose-coloured phaeton, again dressed in rose and in a blue phaeton. Now she is on horseback, another day, in an elegant sea-shell of rock crystal, she drives two sorrel steeds swift as the lightning.

The king's curiosity was roused. He inquired her name, and sent her game from his chase.

She followed His Majesty to the palace of Versailles, and publicly declared her romantic passion. There was great excitement at court, and it amused Louis to keep her hidden for a time, but he soon addressed a letter to her from the front in Flanders, "*A la marquise de Pompadour.*" She had accomplished her ambition. For twenty years she lived in regal magnificence, the real ruler of Louis XV and his court. But they were years of anxiety and intrigue, and at forty she was prematurely old. The king had long tired of her and, after her death, he watched the hearse that was taking her body to Paris, and coolly calculated the time when it would arrive at its destination.

But here we are in the Pompadour station! As the train came in, the pretty American nurses who had come over with us from the monastery waved us goodbye, and we were off once more for Paris. We sat up all night in a compartment, and it was very cold, but we got into town in time for a nice little breakfast in my rooms at the Ritz.

Of course, as usual, I ran from pillar to post after my papers; but this time I had company, for two of Mrs. Daly's nurses were going home with me.

We left Paris one April day—quiet, deserted Paris, with sandbags about its monuments, few taxis, and many closed theatres. Being lucky enough to have a compartment to ourselves, we passed the time by lighting our lamps and making some chocolate. It was a pretty ride as the train poked along toward the coast. The cherry trees were in blossom, and the green fields and red-roofed houses were gay and picturesque.

The northern coast of France, which is part Norman, part Breton, is full of historical interest. Brittany is:

A land of granite, of mighty oaks, and of Druidical remains; land of silence . . . land of a terrible coast, dotted with mysterious Celtic sphinxes; land of poetry and romance of the Middle Ages . . . filled with legend and superstition.

In sharp contrast to it is Normandy:

A land of green valleys walled in from the sea by tall cliffs through which rivers have cut their way, and which the waves have hollowed out, leaving stretches of white sand.

At each of the river mouths a seaport town has been built, of which Boulogne, Dieppe, Havre, and Cherbourg are the largest.

The historical interest of Normandy centres, not in the remote past, but in the days of the Northmen and the great number of places associated with William the Conqueror. He breathed his last, deserted by nobles and servants, at Rouen. Our train stopped here on its way, so we got a look at the fountain in the Place de la Pucelle, which commemorates the execution of Jeanne d'Arc, and a glimpse of the city, one of the most noted in France for its architecture.

Havre, the seat of the exiled Belgian Government, was our destination, for we had been invited to stop over here by the Carton de Wiarts to see another institution for the children of No Man's Land. We got out of the car and trudged off, our long blue veils flying in the wind from the sea, our hands filled as usual with suit cases, papers, and tickets.

At the American bureau we found Madame Carton de Wiart, who took us off to a delightful casino, which had been put at the disposal of the Belgian officials. Several members of the Cabinet were there, and we had a good time talking over the old days in Brussels.

Motoring on to Étretat, the well-known watering place, we stopped at the American hospital for British soldiers, situated in a delightful spot between cliffs, overlooking the sea. Many convalescents were sitting about in their blue suits with red ties, and nurses and orderlies were hovering round. Among these was a friend—a charming boy who had volunteered his services. When I asked just what his work was, he laughed and answered that he might be called the butler, as he did the ordering. He took us out to tea at a fascinating old inn with drooping rafters, antique furniture, and quaint prints.

Madame Carton de Wiart's house was at Harfleur, which was the original seaport at the mouth of the Seine. (Havre dates only from the time when the French explorers were planting the flag of their country in Canada.) This house, loaned by the French Government to the Belgian Minister of Justice, M. Carton de Wiart, stood in the centre of a lovely park behind a high wall. Just over the wall rose an exquisite church tower, and through the garden gate I watched a wedding party entering the church as the bells rang out their gay music.

Such a happy family as I found my hosts—the minister so charming, *Madame* so energetic; a sweet eighteen-year-old daughter, a pretty little girl of eight, a nice boy just home from Eton, and a dear baby. The house was filled with flowers and interesting pieces of old furniture.

Madame Carton de Wiart is one of the real women of this war. Her story is well known over there. For distributing Cardinal Mercier's letter, the Boches took this brave woman out of her home in Brussels without any warning and sent her to Berlin as a prisoner. She was not allowed to say goodbye to her family, or to return for clothes, though later a bag was packed and sent to her. In spite of the fact that she was the wife of a Cabinet Minister, she was treated like the other prisoners.

She did not talk much about her experience to me, but only remarked that no doubt it was very good for her character. She was not starved, at any rate, and notwithstanding her eight months' imprisonment, looked in very good physical condition. During this time, she made a French translation of a book by Brand Whitlock.

Madame took me to see another home for frontier children. It was a charming drive, past picturesque thatched cottages, and cows tethered to stakes after the common method of Normandy. This school, too, was in a monastery, and, like Dandier, seemed rather damp. But the children looked healthy, and judging from the makeshift clothes they wore, the institution must have been run economically. There was a department for doing over the things sent from America. For instance, old felt hats were made into slippers. (It had been costing seven dollars in Belgium to have a pair of shoes resoled.) Clothing not suited to the children's needs was sold for their benefit. *Madame* talked to these little people, and they seemed to love her. They, too, sang songs for us and sent messages of gratitude to America.

Late that afternoon, the minister and his wife took us to the steamer which was to cross the Channel, and gave us little presents, waving goodbye as we left the dock.

The sun was setting as our boat glided out of the harbour, passing torpedo destroyers and big camouflaged steamers. Watching the twinkling lights appear on the shore, I was reminded of the night I had left New York, eight months before.

People at home seem to consider crossing the Channel dangerous, but at this time it was practically safe—as safe as anything can be over there. No boat on this line had ever been torpedoed. I had a nice big stateroom all to myself, and slept soundly till we entered the harbour at Southampton.

CHAPTER 13

The Camouflaged Fleet

London in war-time is quite a different London, although at the station there were taxis and small boys to carry our luggage. As usual, the first thing to do was to visit the police, and this time, the Consul, too, for we had to arrange for our passage home and acquire meat tickets as well. As these were for only a week's ration and we had guests for dinner, they were at once used up, but we didn't seem to care and got on very well without the meat.

The hotels were gay with people and music as in peace days, but the servants did not answer the bells unless they felt like it. Bread was given at meals, but no sugar was served. Even saccharine could not be procured in its place as in Paris, so we simply didn't have any until about a week after our arrival sugar suddenly appeared on the break-fast tray. The waiter volunteered the explanation that after a week it was supplied to guests, but I always suspected he gave it or not as his fancy dictated, for he sometimes presented us with matches, but gen-erally did not. Matches were very scarce in London. We were blessed with coal fires and hot baths, however, so what more could we want?

One of our friends, who thought he might allow himself to in-dulge in some favourite dishes at a London restaurant where he had often eaten, told me his experience:—

I went to an old restaurant in Regent Street, with a mind made up for relaxation and a good dinner, and selected a table. First off, the waiter presented me with a miniature dinner card and said that my entire expenditure must limit itself to five shillings, sixpence, including wine. My variety of profanity, however, im-pressed him as unfamiliar, and he relented enough to suggest that, in case I did not belong to His Majesty's forces, I might

144

have what I liked; and then expounded the law with all the ifs, buts, and whereases one becomes familiar with in the study of jurisprudence.

So, I ordered a sole and a partridge roasted with a bread sauce, a dish the place has been famous for since first I knew it. In due time, back he came with the usual 'Very sorry, sir,' but they had weighed every partridge on the premises, and not one was as small as five and one half ounces. So they could not let me have it. I gave up.

Every time I ask for a drink someone tells me that the bar will not be open again for two hours, and of course by that time I have forgotten all about it. I asked to have the fire lighted in my room, but it seems that what I had mistaken for coal were merely the crown jewels painted black to give a cheerful, prosperous look to the room, and I barely escaped a charge for treason. So, I skim through from one day to another, and will be glad enough to get on the boat Saturday if all goes well.

After we had dined one evening with General Biddle, he took us to a concert for overseas men at the Motor Club, where we heard some very good music. The American officers, I know, appreciate such courtesies, which certainly do tend to draw the two countries closer together.

After working at the front, we especially enjoyed the opportunity of going to the theatres. The plays were remarkably good, far better than those in Paris, in fact. They were mostly American in character—with a great many jokes, plenty of pretty girls, good singing and dancing, and superb costumes.

As motors were almost impossible to get, we were grateful to Mrs. Whitelaw Reid for sending us hers, so that we might see what our Red Cross was doing in England and learn something about the British war work.

The American Red Cross headquarters were especially attractive, and the comfortable Nurses' Home nearby was in a lovely old house run by an English woman. It seemed empty just then, but I was told it was often filled.

The American workrooms turned out the very best garments I had seen, made of excellent material. Although most of the workers were volunteers, some of the employees—Belgian women—were paid. The packing-rooms, too, seemed extremely well managed.

Three Red Cross hospitals were visited—Lancaster House, St. Catherine's Lodge, and Baroda House. It appeared that the money which supported these was sent from the United States and there were some American nurses, but most of them were British, and the hospitals were intended for British officers. I was told they would take in ours as well, but at that time they had had very few. The sisters seemed unusually nice. All three establishments were pretty, clean, and homelike—and if one can use a single word for all, that word is *perfect*.

Kitchener House and California House were run economically on the same lines, by an American woman. California House was started at the beginning of the war to teach trades to disabled Belgian soldiers, who were allowed to attend classes there while being treated. Nearly all the trades were taught, even Japanese lacquer-work, and the art of making pictures in inlaid wood. These cripples really produced some beautiful things.

I remember a wood-carver who had just finished a lovely box. When Miss F., who was with me, offered to buy it, to our surprise the man did not seem pleased. Maybe he clung to it because he loved it so much—perhaps feeling the box might be his last effort. Although in reality quite young, the Belgian looked like an old man, for he had been shot to pieces. The doctor did not see how he could possibly live with all his wounds.

In another room a blind soldier, squatting on the floor, selected the lengths he wanted from a bunch of twigs, and turned them into shape, making a rough basket. The poor fellow's complete blindness and his great haste, as if his very life depended on it, made the tears come to my eyes.

At Kitchener House for Tommies the sitting-room overlooked a pleasant garden, and was warmed by an open fire and supplied with many books and magazines and writing materials. In the dining-room there were pretty volunteer waitresses, and flowers on all the tables. The patients were allowed to take their friends there for tea, and it was very popular.

For British war work they showed the hospital supply department, in which the carpenter shop was particularly worthy of notice. It was filled with volunteer workmen, older men of all classes, making crutches, trays, and other hospital articles. In the cellar the boxes were packed, and on the top floor was a canteen.

Perhaps the most interesting British institutions visited were Roe-Hampton and the Orthopaedic Hospital. Three beautiful adjoining

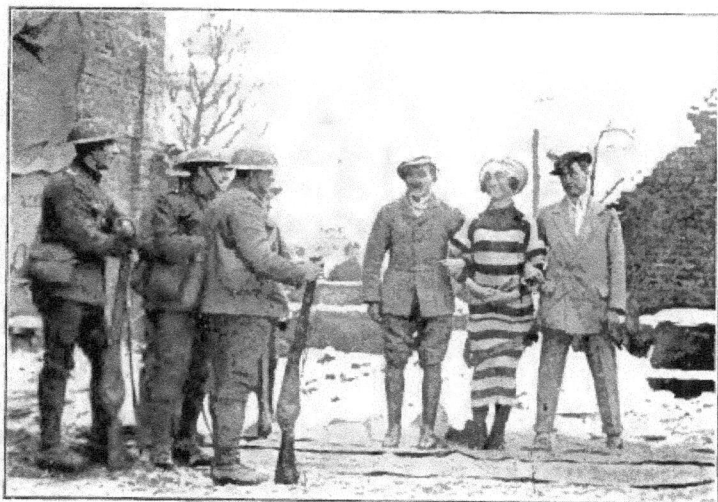

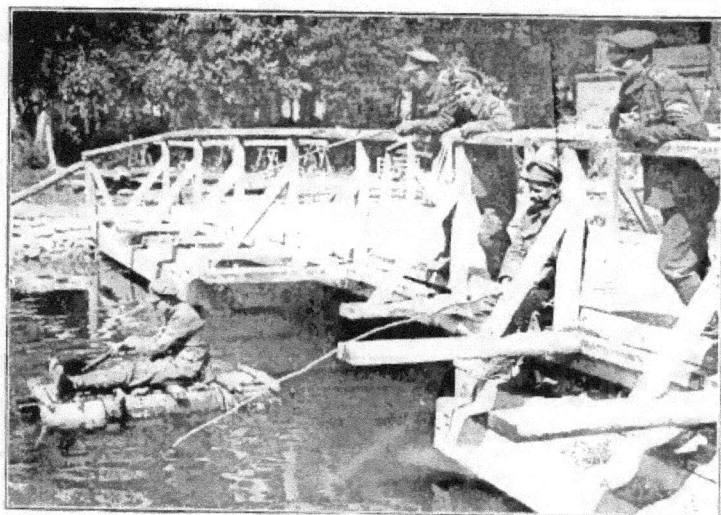

TOMMIES AT PLAY IN FRANCE

estates in the country were given for Roe-Hampton, and barracks were put up in the parks to accommodate the many mutilated soldiers. The place was devoted to fitting on artificial limbs and teaching the soldiers how to use them. It had become a little town in itself, for here, too, all the trades were taught and practiced. Carpenter shops and tailoring establishments were carried on not only to help pay expenses, but also that the soldiers might add to their own slender incomes.

Kitchener House and California House had special permits for trades because they were so small and were run by the American Red Cross, but the men at Roe-Hampton were obliged by the labour unions to continue the trades they had already practiced before the war. The labour question will be hard to adjust in the future when all the wounded come home.

We walked through the workshops and canteen and the wards where the patients slept. Thousands of cripples pass through this institution, generally remaining about three weeks. There were many who had lost both legs, but when I asked the doctor what proportion came with both legs off, he answered, "Less than a third." It appears that a man with one limb cut off below the knee can get on very well indeed. He soon learns to run and even do gymnastics, play tennis and golf. But the man with his leg cut off above the knee finds the artificial one more tiresome and difficult to handle, and he will probably limp. This establishment especially interested me because I had been at work in the operating-room where Dr. Vandervelde made a specialty of cutting off arms and legs.

One doctor was examining a man's stump and fitting it into the half-made artificial leg. A little wood had to be whittled off, so the soldier was told to return in about an hour to have it readjusted. Men with both legs gone were wheeling themselves around in chairs all over the grounds; other cripples were hopping about—some with crutches, some with canes. Still others were trying to manage a newly acquired leg, which at first, they found very troublesome, and could use for only a short time.

The American Hanger leg, made of wood covered with leather, is probably the best for the price. I find it is manufactured in Washington, D.C., and costs (if I remember correctly) about forty dollars, although soldiers may order extra appliances that add to the expense. This limb, like Dr. Depage's, is shaped somewhat like a real leg, but is lighter than the Belgian limb. The French leg I understand is good, but higher priced. The aluminum one has not proved a success. When an artificial leg is dressed with boot and stocking, it can scarcely be distinguished from a natural one, if the man manages it well.

Artificial arms have not been so well perfected, though the kind made in the United States is good. They are certainly all right for a clerk, but unfortunately not strong enough for a labourer. The cripples very often will not take the trouble to learn to use them, making the remaining limb do all the work if possible. The French Coed arm is of the same type as the American. The English have invented a "worker's arm," and gave some remarkable exhibitions with it—one man was digging, and another playing golf. This arm, the doctor stated, had not been entirely perfected, but he felt that it was the thing most needed.

This institution impressed me as greatly worthwhile and one we could well copy In America after the war.

At the other large British hospital—the Orthopaedic—I noticed numbers of baths of different kinds, footbaths with running water for trench feet and delicious bubbly warm baths for the nervous patients. Here were endless electrical machines of all kinds, and rooms for massage. There was one department for nervous patients managed by a marvellous nurse who had made no end of cures, "almost as many as Dr. Worcester in Boston." In one case where the patient had been in bed for a very long time, he walked to the carpenter shop and got a job, after only a few hours of talk and treatment with this nurse. The patient exhibited for us was obliged to walk on a chalk-line for several yards. He had greatly improved, they said—was in fact almost cured. One shoulder had drooped, and for months the doctor could do nothing for him. The man had got the notion that he would never be able to walk upright or in a straight line again, and the doctor told us it was often a fixed idea such as this that prevented a man from being cured. Sometimes a soldier did not want to get well and go back to the trenches.

Word came at last that our ship was about to sail. At nine o'clock one morning we were ensconced in a little compartment and whirled away into the English landscape. It was very beautiful that day, passing through Cheshire and Warwick; through grey meadows divided by rows of hedges; past cottages and lodges almost hidden among the foliage, the chimney-tops with blue smoke curling above them showing where farmhouses stood; across little flowing rivers with rows of willows weeping over them—I had forgotten England was so lovely. Every now and then the train slowed down for a manufacturing town with volumes of black soot pouring forth, but it soon sped out again into the bright country. Even Liverpool looked picturesque as the sun tried to pierce through the brown fog, and the grimy city buildings appeared quite handsome as they stood out on the green parking.

The consul and Colonel Gilmore, old friends, met us at the station in Liverpool and hurried us off in a motor through the crowded streets. The Americans had speeded up things there considerably. Six ships were being loaded then in a day, the time it used to take to fill one—all due to American methods.

Thousands of Yanks were cheering and waving on the troop ships entering the harbour as we went aboard our steamer to sail for home. What a sight it was—this glorious Camouflaged Fleet! There were about fifteen troop ships in the fleet and twelve torpedo destroyers. The latter were painted grey, while the others were all camouflaged.

When I left America in September, I was disappointed in the camouflage of the ships in the harbour of New York. They were mostly painted war grey, so it was a real surprise and delight to see the gay harbour of Liverpool.

Our steamer was painted after the American method—to be as nearly invisible as possible. The colours were in faint pastel shades put on in small squares. When I saw the liner, my first idea was that it had the measles or some strange disease. On second thought I believed it must be carnival-time and that merry-makers had thrown confetti all over it—or could the boat be intended for the comic opera stage?

I was not disappointed on seeing the British camouflaged boats! They exceeded even my wildest dreams. The British idea is not to make the ship invisible, but to deceive as to its direction and length—the bow, for instance, often being painted to represent the stern. They were even sometimes made to look like two boats—unbelievably queer! One had a destroyer under full steam painted on her side. The prominent colours seemed to be green, blue, white, and black; sometimes done in figures, or resembling a Scotch plaid, or squares and triangles, or strange Cubist designs. There were curling, crazy lines—often carried on to the lifeboats, which were painted half and half. These designs are quite incomprehensible to the lay mind. One wonders if some Cubist artist has gone entirely mad—and perhaps the whole world, too.

Our steamer remained in the river over twenty-four hours. Various excuses were given for this delay. The boats were to sail at once into the danger zone and all must be allowed time enough to get ready. The sailors would have to be sobered up and the passengers given a chance to drill with life-belts. (I had bought a life-belt such as the British sailors wear, but was told to put on the ship's belt as well, over it, in case of necessity.) Moreover, our sailing depended on the tides, they said. But probably the real reason for keeping us in the river, was that a big U-boat was known to be out in the Atlantic prowling round.

Passing out of the river, the ships formed a procession, ours being in the centre of four lines, with the torpedo destroyers outside. For some time, a Blimp dirigible balloon hovered over us, diving and leaping like a great silver fish, or, as one man expressed it, "like an animated advertisement for a cigar." From a height one can see far down into the water, so dirigibles are especially good at discovering submarines.

To our astonishment, instead of going toward Queenstown, the liner steamed northward between Ireland and Scotland. The weather was cold, and the water smooth. There was a naval officer on board, who, with engineers and radio men, had a crew of forty under his orders, and a gun forward and aft, but I was informed they seldom saw a periscope and there was not one chance in a thousand of hitting one. Ours was a fast ship, which it is difficult for a U-boat to torpedo, so we felt comparatively safe on that score. But one of the chief dangers of a convoy is a collision while zigzagging in the blackness of the night. After three days we left the camouflaged fleet behind and steamed on alone.

It is not really the duty of the big ship but that of the torpedo destroyer to catch the U-boat. The kind of depth bomb it carries for this purpose is very effective. This simple device has only been used during the past months, but is too dangerous to take on other ships because if there should be a collision it would explode. In the water a depth bomb makes such a terrific explosion that even if it does not hit the submarine it is liable to throw its machinery entirely out of gear. Once a U-boat is discovered, a depth bomb is thrown off over the spot where the submersible has been seen, and the destroyer scuttles away as quickly as possible. Even a boat within two miles can feel the explosion, and the shock to one nearby is so great that sometimes sailors think their own ship has been torpedoed. U-boats are said to travel in fleets.

In answer to my question how one could tell when they had destroyed a submarine, the naval officer said:—

"We rarely have a real sign—sometimes we see wreckage and floating bodies, but not often. In the Destroyer Service it is 'wolf eat wolf.' For instance, in one case three British officers were taken prisoners on a U-boat; a British destroyer knowing this, nevertheless blew up the submersible when it got a chance, although it meant destruction to three British officers, believing it worthwhile in order to get a number of Germans.

"Oh, by the way, have you heard," he asked casually, "that our steamer went within a few feet of a floating mine yesterday? Suppose the sweepers missed it. They're a sporty lot, those mine sweepers, and the chasers with listening devices, and the destroyers and the submarines." Then he turned the talk into other channels.

"Did you see any atrocities in the hospitals at the front?"

I answered, "No; have you seen any?"

"Yes; I saw an American last November in a British hospital who had been crucified, but had been rescued, and was recovering. I have also seen a man who had an eye put out and an arm cut off by a Boche."

I was surprised to hear that the British Navy on the whole had not been as progressive and remarkable as I had imagined. They have not been able to combat the U-boat with any great success until the last few months.

The time passed pleasantly on board. General Alvord, who had been at headquarters with General Pershing, was returning, as well as Mr. Davison, head of the Red Cross, and there were many British reserve officers—captains of merchantmen before the war—on their way to Canada to take back ships. You could tell them by the wavy gold band on the sleeve. It was explained why they still wore buttons on their sleeves—a regulation never changed from olden times, when it was thought necessary to keep the wearer from wiping his nose on his cuff!

They were a bunch of jolly old sea-dogs, those men of the British reserve. One of them told me that he came from Prince Edward Island, and that he had been a policeman, a fireman, and a skipper carrying timber in the Spanish Main. He was thought to have been killed in Halifax at the time of the explosion, and his brother attended his funeral. "But," the old tar laughed, "I turned up again, to the consternation of everybody."

Another character on board was the ship's doctor. While in Mexico he had been put against a wall three times to be shot, had sailed on a ship that was torpedoed in the Mediterranean, and had experienced other thrilling adventures. There were besides several men who had been on a torpedoed ship not once but twice.

At the table sat some American destroyer men, one of whom, because of my interest in the navy, gave me his journal. Since a destroyer which is taking part in the war is named Perkins after my father, I read this officer's journal with special appreciation, while we zigzagged homeward through the fog, and think it may not be out of place as the closing chapter of this book.

CHAPTER 14

"It's A Great Life"

There's a roll and pitch and a heave and hitch
To the nautical gait they take.
For used to the cant of the decks aslant
As the white-toothed combers break
On the plates that thrum like a beaten drum.
To the thrill of the turbines' might,
As the knife bow leaps through the yeasty deeps
With the speed of a shell in flight.

There's a lusty crowd that is vastly proud
Of the slim black craft they drive.
Of the roaring flues and the humming screws
Which make her a thing alive.
They love the lunge of her surging plunge
And the murk of her smoke screen, too,
As they sail the seas in their dungarees,
A grimy Destroyer Crew.

Destroyer Men, by Bert Braley

"*It's a great life if you don't weaken.*" All destroyer men know that saying and it has to them a world of meaning.

The big event had happened. The United States had declared a state of war with Germany, and the eyes of those who knew were turned toward the destroyers. They at least would see active service and very soon.

The main destroyer force was with the Atlantic battleship fleet at its anchorage somewhere on the Atlantic Coast. The message which meant so much came over the radio from Washington on the afternoon of April 6th:—

To Pennsylvania Atlantic Fleet
The President signed an act which declares that a state of war exists between United States and Germany. Acknowledge twenty-five U.S.S.W——, Boston.

April 24—1917

At five o'clock on the afternoon of this day six long, low, grey destroyers, fully equipped and loaded with ammunition, torpedoes, stores, and supplies for overseas duty, slipped their mooring lines and backed out into the stream. In column, one after the other, they stood down the bay, with secret orders to be opened when at a certain point at sea. None on board knew where we were going, but it was the secret belief of every one that the war zone was to be our destination. So—with less than half a dozen people on the dock to see us off, with no waving of handkerchiefs or blowing of whistles—the first expeditionary force, or fighting unit, of the United States quietly put out to sea and headed eastward.

Our secret orders when opened directed us to proceed to a port in the British Isles; to steam in formation under command of the senior destroyer. So, at last we were on our way and our work was indeed cut out for us.

May 4

We have arrived. It has been too rough to touch this log since the day we left the other side. We have had eight days of continuous bad weather, when life on board has been a burden and the W has appeared more like a submarine than a surface craft. Our speed has been slow to economize on fuel. Eating from the wardroom table became so hazardous that we gave it up, preferring to brace ourselves on the transoms and hold the plates and bowls on our laps. Imagine a small vessel drawing nine or ten feet of water, with beam thirty feet and three hundred and fifteen feet long, being tossed about in the waves like a cork for nine or ten days! I have not had my clothes off during this time, and have slept wherever I could find a dry place for my mattress. My room, in the very bow of the ship, was almost untenable in a sea-way, due to the motion. And seasickness! A man is a marvel who has never been sick on a destroyer.

Yes, this has been a sobering trip for all of us in a way, and has made us realise that we are up against a grim, hard campaign of anti-submarine warfare. The hardest and most discouraging of all, I believe.

Well out to sea we were met by the British destroyer *Mary Rose*

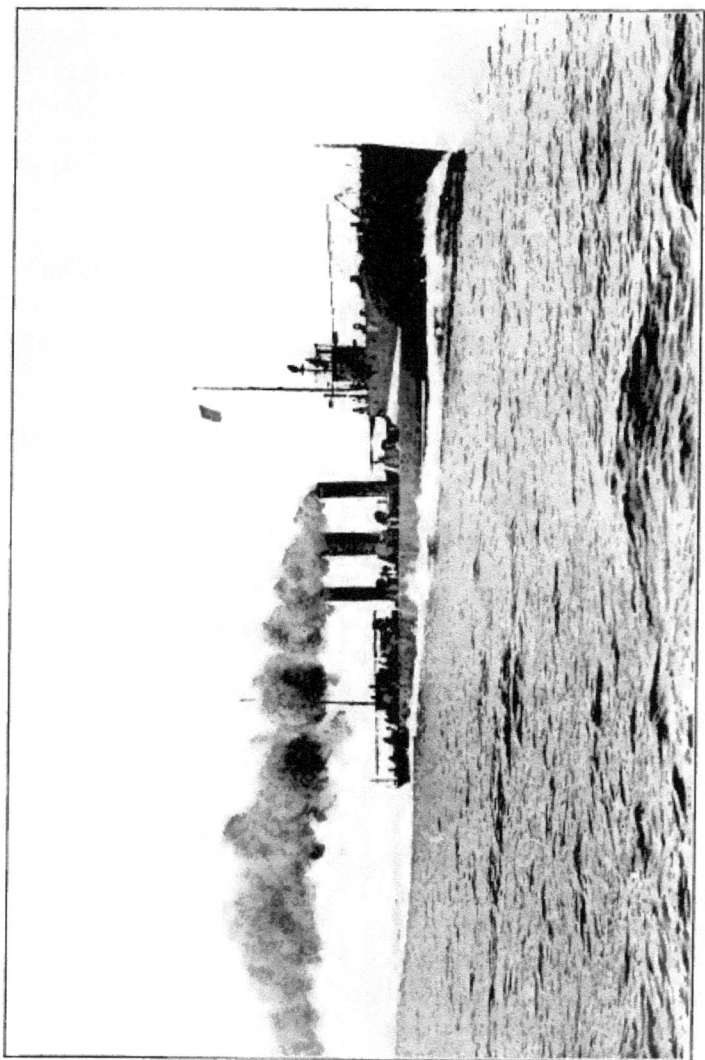

UNITED STATES DESTROYER PERKINS

and escorted to our destination. (The *Mary Rose* was afterwards sunk with all hands in the North Sea by a German raider.) We were given a splendid welcome by the people, and in the evening met many of the British army and navy officers.

When Admiral Bayly, R.N., asked our division commander when our destroyers would be ready for sea he seemed greatly surprised when the answer was, "As soon as we can take on fuel and water, sir."

And so, the first division of American destroyers joined the British forces under command of Admiral Sir Lewis Bayly, and started on the long months of fighting the Hun submarine. The incidents of action are many and thrilling. A periscope sighted—the general alarm—a dash over the spot, and in five minutes all is over. Sometimes a long time passes before another chance of attack.

The German submarine is *good*. He is up to every trick known to the trade—and the odds always seem to be in his favour so long as he has no mishaps to his machinery.

Destroyer men are constantly on the alert. That theirs is a nerve-racking business there is no question, and instant decision is necessary in almost every case. Usually we are at sea from twenty to twenty-five days per month, and when at first put to work on this schedule we wondered which would hold out the longest, the ships or their personnel. But as time went on and the ship kept on "moting" without a break, the crews toughened up and hardened without realising it.

The Navy Department furnished us with fleece-lined coats and the warmest clothes that could be found. It was absolutely necessary that we should be warm—and dry—and well fed. We have been all three, and the spirit of the men I believe to be the best of any branch of any navy in the world. A rough, hard week at sea, when sleep has been scarce and food none too palatable, due to difficulty in cooking, is at once forgotten upon returning to port, and scarcely a growl is heard when ordered to sea again in thirty-six or forty-eight hours.

May 12

This morning sighted a lifeboat floating high out of water with mast shipped—she was adrift. We ranged up alongside of it to see if anyone was inside—just before closing it we increased speed to twenty-two knots, and as we passed a torpedo was fired close under our stern. The boat was a bait placed there by a German submarine in the hope that some unsuspecting vessel would stop, believing survivors were inside.

This afternoon we passed through a great deal of wreckage—a dead mule, dead pig, numerous bales and boxes, once in a while a boat upright or capsised, many spars and hatches.

Today we intercepted radio that another division of American destroyers had arrived, also that our arrival on the 4th has been announced by the British Admiralty. That means the U.S. papers will tell our people at home where we are.

July 1.

We have just finished escorting our first convoy of American troops to France. Things are looking up! When we put to sea, we did not know the Americans had any troops within three thousand miles. It was a big surprise and a joyful one to find that our soldiers were really started. As we ranged alongside to take our position on the flank the khaki-clad army files which lined the rails of the huge ships certainly looked as good to us as we must have looked to them. The first to enter the French port was an army transport, the second was loaded with marines. I wonder who the two marines were who jumped overboard in the channel and swam ashore, in order to keep the tradition of the service—"*The Marines, always the first to land.*"

July 10

Captain T., of the Royal Irish, told me today of their new daughter of the regiment, and the part played by the U.S. Destroyer *C——* in their getting her.

A lifeboat was sighted at sea. Upon steaming past at high speed to investigate, it was found that a little child was sitting up in the middle of the boat between two men lying in the bottom. The *C——* circled round it and went alongside. Two sailors were lowered over the side on a line. The men in the boat were found to be dead. Evidence showed that they were Norwegian sailors, but no clue was found as to the name of their vessel or where they were from. The men were buried at sea and the little girl taken on board. She was about two years old and in perfect health, warmly dressed, and her clothing was of the best. She seemed perfectly happy.

In her little pockets were several sea biscuits and some dried fruit. The men had starved to death, leaving the child their food. She was landed at the post of Captain T.'s company and put in his charge. The child was a perfect little beauty, and cheerful every minute. The regiment has sworn that she shall have the best the country can offer, and that they will never give her up.

July 14

Great excitement at Admiralty House. U.S. Destroyers *D*—— and *B*—— ordered to proceed immediately to latitude —— and longitude —— and pick up survivors of U.S. Destroyer *McD*——.

Two merchant ships, one with wireless and one with a single gun, meet up with each other in the war zone and decide to proceed together for mutual protection. The *McD*——, unknown to ship with wireless, had been sent out to escort her; before she arrived, ship with one gun had been sunk. Merchantman with radio sent out message:

> My escort torpedoed—sunk.

Admiralty House, believing this referred to Destroyer *McD*——, sent out as stated the *D*—— and *B*—— under full speed to pick up the *McD*——'s survivors.

Later the *McD*—— intercepting message, but missing her own name, sent in message to Admiral ——:

> Am in position searching for survivors!

I have just been detached from the *W*—— to another destroyer, the *B*——. Being a reserve officer I have to get acquainted all over again, but this is easy in the war zone. Was sorry at first, but am glad now. The *B*—— is a fine vessel with a keen set of officers. Reserves at present are rather scarce on destroyers.

July 20

Escorting British merchantman *N*——. Sea smooth, clear weather. At 5.30 p.m. Ensign H. called down from the bridge, "Convoy torpedoed." A rush to general quarters (battle stations), thirty knots on the engines, and we began circling the sinking ship. No submarine was ever seen. The torpedo, which passed three hundred yards astern of us, struck the *N*—— in her forward hold just forward of the boilers. She was loaded with ore and started down at once. One boat was smashed by the explosion, leaving but one other. This was immediately lowered and her crew of twenty-eight all escaped. The chief engineer was the only person injured.

The engines were never stopped, so she kept on surging ahead. Her bow settled lower and lower, until the swells began breaking over her. In an incredibly short time, her bow went under, her stern shot high in the air one third of her length out of water—smoke poured out of her stack, her propeller still turned over, and in this position, she took her final plunge to the bottom of the sea. This is but a poor description of what is really only too common a sight in the war zone. But never so common but that it leaves one breathing hard and appalled by the awful destructiveness of the Hun torpedo.

The captain of the N—— was a cheery English skipper, very cool and always smiling—his most vicious remark was, "Drat the fellow, I was almost home!" We kept the men on board two days, all of which time these merchant sailors were thoroughly seasick. Oh, these destroyers!

August—

The U.S. destroyers O—— and C—— , while in port loading stores and making minor repairs, received urgent orders from Admiralty House to proceed to sea immediately to attack submarine sighted on surface at a certain point. The O—— put to sea one half-hour after receiving these orders and was followed an hour later by the C——.

The British admiral commanding sent the following message to the O——:—

Flag to O——
Congratulate you on quick work in putting to sea. (1130)

Later:—

O—— to Flag
Returning to port. Machinery defect. (1350)

Flag to O——
Cancel my 1130. (1430)

September 12

At sea with division of destroyers, one of which, the C—— , stopped to pick up a boat with survivors. The radio intercepted from C—— to Flag was:

Picked up boat with five survivors from the British Chinese S.S.
V—— , torpedoed and sunk Sept. 10th.

The story that goes with this is one the German submarine service should be proud of.

The V—— was sunk without warning and her captain taken on board the submarine a prisoner. The submarine then shelled the lifeboats with shrapnel. The chief engineer had both legs cut off above the knees. The first officer had shell pass through his chest. Others were wounded and killed. The one boat which was left, the one picked up by the C——, had in it six men, five Chinese and one white man, three others in it having died of wounds. The five Chinese were taken on board, but the man in the stern would not move. He sat upright, apparently in good health, but with a dazed expression on his face, and would make no effort to rise or speak. When ordered to come on board, he suddenly, without the slightest warning, toppled over the side and sank like a stone.

The five Chinese were very suspicious and would not touch the whiskey offered them until they were finally convinced that their rescuers were not Germans, but Americans.

September 15
The H.M.S. M—— , a sloop, based with us, was torpedoed while on patrol near us and three men killed. She was taken into port under tow. The German submarine commander sent the following message to Admiral B. at Admiralty House:—

Send out some more sloops—we like them.

I have been acting at intervals as ship's censor. It is not popular duty by a long way, but it has its recompense if one has a sense of humour. I am eagerly following the love affairs of a certain one of our quartermasters. He has three violent ones on hand at the present writing—faithful to all. I am betting on "blue eyes."

We have one little sailor as bad as they make them, always in trouble both on ship and on shore. But he writes his sweetheart over home not to fail to send him all her Sunday-School lessons! He is a little rascal, but I am in great hopes these lessons will make him a better boy. I also know that a girl back home has two sweethearts on the same ship—this ship—and they both fill their letters full of slander about each other.

I notice two types of men writing to their wives—one writes loving letters, shrieking of "her" day and night, on ship and shore, etc., but rarely encloses a check. On the other hand, the fellows who write, "I take my pen in hand to let you know that I am well and hope you are the same," usually slip in twenty dollars or so. Less words, more money.

Of course, the censor officer must keep all this to himself, and cannot share his fun with the mess. It is sometimes almost a pity.

October 5
Bound for a port in England for a ten days' refit and five days' leave

for every officer and man. This comes to us about once every five months and is the only break in this life of ours—our only chance to go to a theatre or a party, or see new faces.

Yes, this is a big event for us, these five days in London, and the man who says London is dull in war-time never came from a destroyer on five days' leave after five months at sea with British weather.

At 5, Cavendish Square, London, within easy distance of many of the theatres, shops and hotels of that huge city, is situated "The American Officers' Inn."

This inn is to the American officers what the Eagle Hut is to the enlisted men. Although entirely separate, both are run by the Y.M.C.A.

The inn is an old English residence fronting on Cavendish Square, one of London's many little open parks. It has sleeping accommodations for about forty officers, though meals can be served to many more.

By the use of a huge knocker on the door you can gain admittance, and find yourself at once in the large front hall, in the midst of an atmosphere of cordiality. This is really a lounge, with an open fireplace, large, deep chairs, a table, and a telephone exchange board with a pretty London girl operating it—a voluntary worker. At the table you will find Mrs. Nichols ably presiding as chaperon and voluntary secretary. She has a son, an officer in the navy, but is also considered as a mother by every young fellow who is fortunate enough to put up at this delightful place. She meets you with a welcoming smile, and in a moment, you have shaken hands with those standing about, old friends in many cases.

Here you find a scattering of officers of all branches and corps of the army and navy, some on leave, some *en route* to France. Flyers, doctors, marine corps, and coast-guard officers, battleship and destroyer men—you join them and accept a cigarette, and in a moment your back to the fireplace and are puffing out long puffs of smoke and taking part in the gossip of the hour—with an eager ear for events back home.

On the ground floor are the library and writing-room, dining- and serving-rooms. A wide staircase on the side leads to the floors above. I was shown to my room—the last one available—by another charming English girl.

With one or two exceptions, all the work at the inn is done by voluntary workers. A number of London's nicest girls volunteer to do the work, to make it a success and cut down expenses. These young ladies take turns or watches—one will come on say from 7 a.m. to noon on four days a week; next week she will have the afternoon watch, another week the evening. Their work consists of waiting on table, doing the cooking, washing dishes, sweeping, dusting, making beds, standing a door watch, and many other things which mean hard work. It is good hard work, too, as anyone who has been there can testify. And the chances are when not on duty at the inn these girls are working at some canteen or hospital, in all putting in eight or ten hours of war work daily, without pay.

I was informed there was to be a dance that night. Would I come? "Gladly!" The ballroom is on the second floor, with an alcove at one end to take a real sure-enough American billiard and pool table. This was constantly in use, even during the dance, with other chaps standing around smoking before the open fireplaces. Although a few young ladies from outside were invited, they were mostly workers at the inn who had shifted from the uniform of the day to evening dress—and it seemed as though all the loveliness in London was there. A Naval Flying Corps officer played the piano, a doctor played the *mandolin*, and the party was perfect. The nearest thing to a large house party that I could think of.

At breakfast next morning (as late as you wish up to eleven) you will probably find the smart young waitress who approaches you with your coffee and porridge to be the same girl who, the night before, gave you those three or four good dances. Only she was up and at work at 7.30 a.m. while you have just eased in at 10.30.

But an officer who has interests outside or is too busy to avail himself of all that is going on at the Inn is in no way bound to stay there—this is simply his hotel or club, where expenses are in all ways reduced to the minimum. The inn is to each officer just what he wishes to make it.

Many of the theatres send complimentary stalls to the inn for officers who care to use them.

Many invitations to other things are sent to the officers here, so it is rare that one has nothing to do.

The result of all this is that the evils of London night life lose all their charms in the face of this, our London home.

October 15

At sea again and our work continues as before. We have all had a big change and a good rest.

The admiral believes that as the *B——* has just been overhauled she is good for even a little stiffer pace than before—and I am sure the men are in better shape. We now look forward to our next refit period—four or five months hence.

The U.S. Destroyer *C*—— was torpedoed today, our first vessel from this base to be hit by a torpedo since the beginning of the war. I wonder if the word has been passed at Berlin that we have been having too easy a time of it. Two days ago, a merchant ship was sunk off the coast, and the submarine commander told the sailors in the boats that the waters around here had been infested by American destroyers for the past few months, and they had had it pretty easy, but their time would soon come.

He had just taken one prisoner when his lookout reported a destroyer on the horizon, bearing down on them from the northwest. He sang out *"Heraus!"* and after telling those in the boats that it was the American Destroyer *P*—— coming, and that she would pick them up, the hatches were closed, and she submerged. In twenty minutes, the *P*—— took on board all survivors—a proof that the Germans know pretty well where we are at all times.

November 4

The *Army and Navy Register* published the following item:

The Navy Department is informed that the American steamship *Luckenback* was engaged by an enemy submarine on October 19th. The engagement lasted from 7.35 a.m. until 11.40 a.m. and was broken by the arrival of an American patrol boat. The *Luckenback* was hit several times, but no serious damage was done to the ship. Several of the crew of the *Luckenback* and two members of the armed guard were wounded.

We were close by, and although ours was not the rescuing vessel, I joined the *Luckenback* shortly after and saw her shell-riddled hull. We had really followed the fight by radio. The intercepted messages came through the air like this:—

Luckenback to U.S.S. *N*——
Code books overboard. When will you arrive?

N—— to *Luckenback*
Two hours.

Luckenback to *N*——
Look out for boats—shelling us now.

N—— to *Luckenback*
Don't surrender.

Luckenback to *N——*
Never.

That evening we lost the H.M.S. *F——* , a huge merchant cruiser, the ocean escort of our convoy. She was a great loss, and had many people on board. Due to the excellent seamanship on the part of Captain J., of the U.S.S. *C——* , no lives were lost. He put his destroyer up alongside the *F——* and the survivors were taken on board by rope ladders and boat falls. For this he was recommended for the D.S.O. Just as the *C——* shoved off, the big merchant cruiser took her final plunge to the bottom. Through the work of this same *C——* the submarine that had done the damage was struck off the German list for good.

December 10
Yesterday we took on board the *B——* five survivors from the ill-fated Destroyer *Jacob Jones*, torpedoed the afternoon of the 7th. These men, with two others who were left ashore at the Falmouth hospital, were picked up by the S.S. *Catalina* which passed their raft close aboard at eight o'clock the same night. It was pitch black, but the men's shouts were heard on the *Catalina*. At first, she started to leave them, thinking it was one of the usual German submarine traps. But the men's final wail, which was heard as the *Catalina* pulled away, the captain knew came from men's hearts. He stopped his ship and took them on board.

Standing in that icy water up to their waists in those doughnut rafts in December was more than human endurance could bear. Nine men as strong as are in our navy died one at a time inside of four hours, and were slipped over the side by the others—each one of the survivors almost hoping he would be the next and looking forward to the relief that would come when he could finally loosen his hold. This is what happened to one raft—the story of the others is about the same. One officer and seventy men were lost; two prisoners went to Germany on the submarine.

After the explosion, when the ship had gone down, a sailor and the captain came up and struck out together. The spirit of our boys is shown by this sailor's first remark—"Well, captain, where do we go from here?"

That famous snatch of dialogue between an admiral of the old school and the captain who was towing him through the Straits of Gibraltar illustrates what I mean by the destroyer men's spirit:—

Unless the wind and sea abate,
I cannot tow you through the strait.

As long as you have wood and coal,
You'll tow me through, G—d—your soul!

So long as we have wood and coal, the destroyers will be on their job at all costs, zigzagging back and forth over the perilous waters of the Atlantic.

Appendix

CHAPTER 1

General Information for Canteen Workers of W.W.R.C. of
A.R.C. in France
1. Necessary Papers.

(a) French:

1. *Carte d'Identité.*

Present letter from *hôtel* at Police station of that arrondissement.
Must know date of father's and mother's birth and death.

2. *Extrait du Registre d Immatriculation.*

Present *carte d'identité* at *Préfecture de Police*, opposite Notre-
Dame, *Escalier F.*

Note: 5 photographs without hats are required.

(b) American Red Cross Identification Card.

Apply at 4 Place de la Concorde, French Canteen division,
with passport, 2 photographs.

French papers (above) are necessary to secure card, but are not
necessary for application. *Note:*

1. Application for a *Carnet d'Étranger* to enter the war zone is
made *only through the* A.R.C. when the worker has been defi-
nitely assigned by the W.W.R.C. to a post. Worker should then
report the Canteen Division with all official papers and two
photographs. *This Carnet must not be applied for by individual.*

2. Temporary work in Paris to which worker will be detailed is
as important as her permanent work and a careful record will
be kept of it.

2. Uniform.

(*a*) Travelling: (Purchased at Nicoll's, 29 rue Tronchet and 23
rue des Mathurins—Price: *Frs.* 225.)

1. Grey coat and skirt with collar and cuffs of "*horizon bleu*" and letters ARC in red on shoulder straps. Directrices of canteen have shoulder straps of the same shade as collar and cuffs,

2. Grey overcoat with lining to match, or blue.

3. Blouses—Plain tailored blue or white of silk and flannel.

4. Necktie to match blue.

5. Hat: dark grey, with black grosgrain band bordered with same shade of blue. (Purchased at Belle-Jardinière, 2 rue du Pont-Neuf.)

(*b*) Working: (Purchased at Trois Quartiers, Boulevard des Capucines, from Mrs. Burton or Mme. Michel at the Blouse counter.)

1. Blue linen aprons—*Frs.* 19.75 and 15.50.

2. White collar and cuffs—*Frs.* 5 a pair.

3. White *infirmière* veil—*Frs.* 3.25.

3. Miscellaneous.

(*a*) Baggage: a small steamer trunk may be taken to canteens. 30 kgs. allowed *free*; not more than 100 kgs. permitted.

(*b*) Money: American Express checks are most convenient in war zone.

(*c*) Kodaks: Are *not* permitted in war zone.

4. Finances.

For workers receiving expenses please divide accounts as follows on *expense sheets* secured from Canteen Division of A.R.C.

(*a*) A voucher covering all expenses up to date of arriving in Paris.

(*b*) A voucher covering expenses in Paris. This will be presented every Saturday at 2 p.m. at the office of the Canteen Division of the A.R.C.

(*c*) On arriving at a post, a voucher covering expenses to date of leaving Paris and including transportation (if that is due) shall be mailed to the Canteen Division of the A.R.C; and a check will be forwarded at once.

(*d*) On leaving Paris a flat monthly rate of expenses will be determined and this amount will be forwarded each month from Paris to the individual.

General Requirements for Women Applicants in Red Cross
Service Abroad

1. Must have robust health, certified to after examination by physician designated by Red Cross.

2. Must be free from all German or Austrian connections by birth or marriage.

3. Must not have husband, father, or son in United States Army or Navy at home or abroad.

4. Must be willing to sign contract for one year's service (six months for full volunteers in Canteen Service) in France, Belgium, or Italy, wherever assigned.

5. Must be vaccinated for smallpox and inoculated against typhoid, and paratyphoid, before final acceptance.

6. Must give three references (four in case of Social Service), American citizens, not relatives—one, at least, a woman—who can vouch for applicant's character and ability.

7. In general, applicants should be capable of hard and continuous physical labour under uncomfortable conditions. No woman not ready to give full-time and conscientious service need apply. Good temper, discretion, and self-reliance are also essential. Seriousness of purpose, dignity of deportment are required.

Special Requirements

Social Service: Age 28-50 years. Must speak French or Italian well. Must have training in Social Service or equivalent in experience. Must wear uniform on duty. Must serve for expenses and small salary, or as volunteers.

Canteen Service: Age 25-35 years. Knowledge of French useful. Experience in cooking useful. Must be exceedingly strong and ready for constant hard work. Must wear uniform on duty. It is preferred that Canteen Workers pay their own expenses, but persons who are well qualified are accepted and their expenses paid.

Hospital Hut: Age 25-35 years. Knowledge of French useful. Must wear uniform on duty. Must have ability to make a pleasant, homelike recreation centre. Music, ability to read aloud well and to organise entertainments are important assets. Must serve as volunteers or for expenses.

Clerical Service: Age 28-40 years. Knowledge of French useful. Certificate of professional proficiency will be required and test may be given if necessary. Clerical workers receive a sum sufficient to cover living expenses, and transportation is paid by the Red Cross.

Nurses' Aids: Age 25-35 years. Knowledge of French very important. Must be graduates of Red Cross Course in Elementary Hygiene and Home Care of Sick, or must agree to take course at once. Must be recommended by instructor. Hospital experience valuable. Must be exceedingly strong and ready for constant hard work. Must wear uniform on duty. Must serve as volunteers or for expenses.

CHAPTER 2

Rules for Canteen Workers

1. Do not ask the soldiers any military questions—where they are going or what happened at their last post.

2. Do not write about such facts; above all, do not criticize anything French in any way. Every letter is read by the military authorities, who are specially interested in the tone of American communications.

3. Do not "*tutoyer*" the soldiers, nor call them "*petit.*" The French object to it. Always address them as "*Monsieur.*"

4. Do not dispute any question with a soldier who has had too much to drink, no matter how right you are. If necessary, let him go without paying. Any other policy is dangerous.

5. Do not go alone to any military bureau; always take one of your companions with you if there is any business to transact.

6. Do not stand and talk to groups of soldiers outside the Canteen.

7. Do not make appointments to walk or accompany a Frenchman anywhere alone. It is entirely contrary to French customs.

8. Do not do anything in or out of the Canteen to make it conspicuous. The whole town is ceaselessly observing you.

9. Do not forget to greet your French fellow-workers both on their arrival at and their departure from the Canteen. They attach the greatest importance to these little acts of courtesy.

10. Do not fail to be guided by their preferences as far as is consistent with the efficiency of the Canteen service.

11. Don't fail to be *quiet* and courteous in the houses where you

may be lodged.

12. Do not fail to remember that you are on duty in the War Zone and that you are not in France for sight-seeing.

13. Do not forget that uniforms are made to be worn, and can only be laid aside with the permission of the Directrice of your Unit or by the special order of the Central Committee.

14. Do not fail to see that your "*Carnet d'Étranger*" is stamped by the proper authorities both on your arrival at your destination and on your departure.

Here are a few phrases we were asked to learn. These give an idea of our work.

Canteen Phrase Book

1.	Achetez vos billets au guichet.	1. Buy your tickets at the desk.
2.	A gauche.	2. To the left.
3.	A droite.	3. To the right.
4.	Un peu plus loin.	4. A little farther on.
5.	Devant vous.	5. In front of you.
6.	La monnaie.	6. Change.
7.	Avez-vous de la monnaie à me rendre?	7. Have you change to give me?
8.	Vous n'avez pas de sous?	8. Have you not any pennies? ·
9.	Demandez la monnaie à un camarade.	9. Ask a comrade for change.
10.	Allez chercher la monnaie à la caisse.	10. Go to the desk for change.
11.	Un sou.	11. One cent.
12.	Un petit sou.	12. One cent.
13.	Un gros sou.	13. Two cents.
14.	Une pièce de 5 sous.	14. A five-cent piece.
15.	Vingt-cinq centimes.	15. Twenty-five centimes.
16.	Une pièce de 10 sous.	16. A ten-cent piece.
17.	Cinquante centimes.	17. Fifty centimes.
18.	Donnez-moi 2 sous pour la consigne du couvert.	18. Give me 2 cents on deposit for forks and spoon.
19.	Le déjeuner commence à dix heures et demie.	19. Lunch is served at half-past ten.
20.	On sert le dîner à cinq heures.	20. Dinner is served at five o'clock.
21.	Qu'est-ce que vous désirez manger?	21. What do you want to eat?
22.	Du bouillon.	22. Bouillon.
23.	De la soupe.	23. Soup.
24.	Du potage.	24. Soup.
25.	Des œufs sur le plat.	25. Fried eggs.
26.	Des œufs durs.	26. Hard-boiled eggs.
27.	Du pain.	27. Bread.
28.	De la viande (or, in poilu slang, singe).	28. Meat.
29.	Du bœuf mode.	29. Beef mode.

30. Un rôti de bœuf.	30. Roast-beef.
31. Bifteck.	31. Beefsteak.
32. Du veau.	32. Veal.
33. Du mouton.	33. Mutton.
34. Du hachis.	34. Hash.
35. Un ragoût.	35. Stew.
36. Du saucisson.	36. Sausage.
37. Du jambon.	37. Ham.
38. Des légumes.	38. Vegetables.
39. Des carottes.	39. Carrots.
40. Du chou.	40. Cabbage.
41. Des navets.	41. Turnips.
42. Des oignons.	42. Onions.
43. Des pommes de terre.	43. Potatoes.
44. Des pommes de terre frites.	44. Fried potatoes.
45. Des pommes de terre sautées.	45. Sautées potatoes.
46. Des légumes secs.	46. Dried vegetables.
47. Des haricots secs.	47. Dried beans.
48. Des pois secs.	48. Dried peas.
49. Des lentilles.	49. Lentils.
50. De la salade.	50. Salad.
51. Des fruits.	51. Fruit.
52. Du fromage.	52. Cheese.
53. Une pomme.	53. An apple.
54. Une orange.	54. An orange.
55. Des raisins.	55. Grapes.
56. Un entremets.	56. Pudding.
57. Des pruneaux.	57. Prunes.
58. Des figues.	58. Figs.
59. La vaisselle.	59. Dishes.
60. Un plateau.	60. A tray.
61. Un bol.	61. A bowl.
62. Une assiette.	62. A plate.
63. Une fourchette.	63. A fork.
64. Un couteau.	64. A knife.
65. Une cuillère.	65. A spoon.
66. Du café (jus).	66. Coffee.
67. Du café au lait.	67. Coffee with **milk**.
68. Du chocolat.	68. Chocolate.
69. Du thé.	69. Tea.
70. Un quart.	70. A tin cup.
71. Voulez-vous attendre le repas complet?	71. Do you want to wait for the meal?
72. On commence à servir à dix heures.	72. We begin to serve at ten o'clock.
73. Le menu consiste de . . .	73. The menu is composed of . . .
74. Il n'y en a plus.	74. There is no more of it.
75. Il n'y a plus de . . .	75. There is no more . . .
76. Essuyez les tables, s'il vous plaît.	76. Please wipe off the tables.
77. Rapportez la vaisselle.	77. Bring back the dishes.
78. Mettez la vaisselle sur le plateau.	78. Put the dishes on the tray.
79. Ramassez les bols.	79. Gather up the bowls.
80. Le dortoir est juste en face.	80. The sleeping quarters are just opposite.
81. Traversez la rue.	81. Cross the street.

82. Vous trouverez les couvertures dans le dortoir.	82. You will find blankets in the sleeping quarters.
83. Les lavabos sont à côté.	83. The wash-room is alongside.
84. Laissez passer les autres, s'il vous plait.	84. Allow the others to pass, please.
85. Avancez un peu.	85. Move on a little.
86. Faites de la place.	86. Make room.
87. Allez dans la salle de récréation.	87. Go into the recreation room.
88. Voilà des cartes-postales.	88. There are postcards.
89. Voilà du papier à lettre.	89. Here is writing paper.
90. La boîte à lettre est dehors.	90. The letter box is outside.
91. Il fait beau temps.	91. It is fine weather.
92. Il fait mauvais temps.	92. It is bad weather.
93. Voulez-vous un petit drapeau américain?	93. Do you want a little American flag?
94. Bonsoir, Monsieur, dormez bien.	94. Good night, sir, sleep well.
95. C'est gratuit, Monsieur.	95. It is free, sir.

A Typical Letter to a Marraine

Ma chère bonne marraine:—

Combien je suis heureux d'avoir fait votre connaissance; je suis tout heureux de vous appartenir comme filleul de guerre; je suis le zouave; vous vous rappellerez bien de moi, puisque vous m'avez accepté comme filleul.

Ma chère marraine, il est dimanche, aussi aujourd'hui nous ne travaillons pas et de l'affaire je m'ennuie passablement, aussi je me permets de venir bavarder un peu avec vous pour dissiper un peu le spleen. Hélas, ce soir à la nuit, je vais placer des fils de fer en avant de notre tranchée avec quelques hommes; voilà déjà quelques nuits que j'en place; et vous pouvez croire que c'est triste de placer ce fil de fer barbelé, on s'accroche les mains à tout instant et on risque aussi k recevoir une balle dans la tête; aussi nous faisons le moins possible de potins pour ne pas se faire entendre par les bodies.

Je vous joins ma photo; laquelle vous fera bien plaisir, puisque je vous l'avais promise mais je suis habillé en civil, et suis en compagnie de mon épouse et de ma petite fille chérie. Je souhaite pour vous, chere marraine, que vous réussissiez pleinement dans toutes vos entreprises de même que votre honorable famille que je n'ai pas l'avantage de connaitre mais pour laquelle je formule les meilleurs de mes voeux.

Vous priant de bien vouloir recevoir l'assurance des meilleurs sentiments de votre respectueux et affectueux filleul qui ne salt comment vous exprimer sa reconnaissance.

173

Tous mes respects,

Ferdinand Ollier caporal
Vous m'excuserez si ma feuille de papier est tachée, car il est rare, c'est comme le tabac. A bientôt de vos bonnes nouvelles.

Extract from Red Cross Bulletin

Through the Bureau of Investigation and Relief Service 105,551 pairs of socks containing shoe laces and candy were distributed at Christmas.

The Bureau of Metropolitan Canteens gave the French soldiers 12,000 comfort kits, 144,000 mirrors and 5000 handkerchiefs.

Christmas celebrations were held in the L.O.C. canteens and gifts distributed to the soldiers. At Châlons, to cite one case, there were two Christmas trees in the big main room. A small stage was set up, and the soldiers sang and recited. The American women workers sang the Star-Spangled Banner. The mass of *poilus* swept their hats off with one movement and cheered. It was a moving spectacle, and the soldiers showed clearly how much our canteen workers have done in the past months to bring home to them the spirit of America.

Letter from a Worker in The Canteen at Châlons during the Spring Drive

You have probably heard of our two weeks of—Hell—no other word describes it—but we have all come through so far, and the Canteen is still serviceable and open, even if a bit the worse for wear.

Our life has been a difficult one. We crawl in the wine cellars in the hills at night—with the whole town for bed companions—a dark, dirty place, but safe. After a sleepless night we venture out at four a.m. to open the Canteen, work madly to feed our cold and hungry men, snatch a bit of food ourselves, take a short nap in any possible corner. Back to the *caves* at dusk. Most of our original rooms are uninhabitable, even if we dared to sleep there, so you see we are really running the Canteen under difficulties.

But we do run it, and the Boches have not gained a thing by their evil attacks—they have killed lots of women, old men and babies, but not a soldier here yet, and have not done any irreparable damage to military things, the beasts! No words can tell what I feel after seeing dear Châlons so mistreated.

A Letter from Miss Katherine Ten Eyck Lansing to her Brother, the Secretary of State

France, Thursday, June 6, 1918.

Long before you receive this you will have received the cable-gram, we hope reached you through the ambassador, and have been relieved of your anxiety about us. We have been living through thrilling days and I am still tired enough to be afraid that I won't write a very clear letter. This is the first chance either of us has had to write, for we have been tremendously busy. Of course, the first news we had of the big German attack came a week ago, Monday. We knew that it was all along the line near us, but felt no anxiety about our own situation, although two of the ladies had decided to go to Paris that day for the day—but decided not to, as they were afraid there might be some difficulty about getting back to —— (a place about twelve miles from the front) on account of the movement of troops. The troops passed all day and we knew they were being taken to the different points of attack.

Tuesday morning there was some excitement in the hall while I was still in bed. I got up to see and found Miss E—— (head of the Canteen) had received a letter from an English friend, couched in very ambiguous terms, but by reading between the lines we made out that he thought we should all go, at once, to Paris, while "the going was still good" as he put it. After consultation with the military authorities we decided there was no immediate danger. Tuesday the ambulances kept going by with the wounded, and Tuesday night Miss E—— took one person and went to see if there was anything to be done at the Evacuation Hospital. We did not all go, as she was not willing. About ten she came back for five more people. Emma could not go, as she was on night duty in the Canteen, but I went with four others, and I never spent such a strange night. As soon as I reached the hospital I was asked if I would go into one of the barracks where the more lightly wounded were and interpret between the French doctors and English.

The hospital is a huge place with wooden shacks for the different wards, and spreads over a great deal of ground. I was taken into one of these barracks crowded with people, becoming more crowded as the night went on. There were both English and French, and I was asked to take the names of all the English, their regiments, enlistments, and so on, and find out where they were wounded. I was told what to do, then left alone, and there I was all night, the room crowded with French, Algerians, Blacks, and English.

As the night wore on the poor things lay down as they could on the floors, under the tables and on the tables, bloody bandages all around. I had made out all the English papers by about half-past two. In the midst of it about one, we had an air raid and I can tell you the bombs never sounded so loud as they did out there, all alone with all those wounded men. In the midst of it someone opened the door and called "*à l'abri*," and those who were able left the shack and went to the *abri*. I went out to see how it was and found many of them standing outside, as the *abri* was full. About four it began to be light and I wondered whether the others had gone home, but as I was alone with all these men I did not like to leave.

A little later some of the officials came in—and then began the task of fitting the papers to the men and getting them off in the train. They wanted me to stay to read the names as they were so difficult to pronounce. I made another list of men who had to go off on stretchers, told the doctors, in French, where they were wounded and so on, and did not get back to the house until twelve at noon. It was rather a long stretch from ten the night before—especially as I had nothing to drink or eat.

In the afternoon I went to the Canteen. Some of the people in —— were beginning to leave and the inhabitants were all gathered in knots around the street. The military movement through the town was something amazing. Of course, excitement ran high. We spent all our days and nights—until Saturday night—at the hospital, with only two people left at the Canteen.

I can't tell you anything about it—only with the most vivid imagination. I do not think anyone can dream of such suffering, such patience, such heroism, or such terrible human wreckage, and until one has seen it they cannot know what war means. We found more than we could do even with our lack of knowledge, giving the men water, washing their bloody faces, interpreting between the English and the French doctors, and wishing we could go a hundred times as fast. One French boy I brought water to and the tears rolled down his face, he had waited so long for it—and for a French boy to cry like that means more than other nationalities.

I have found that you can bear seeing the most horrible wounds if you are doing something. I was so afraid I would not have the courage, but when I was doing something, I did not think of that side of it. I went into the operating-room—or, rather, the room where the wounds were cleansed and dressed—and gave water to the men on the tables, but the hardest thing was to give milk or water to the men whose faces were completely smashed to pieces. No words could describe such sublime endurance of suffering.

Friday night we had a heavy air raid. Miss E——, Miss L——, and I were in bed and were caught in the house before we could go to the *cave*, and I must say we were all pretty scared, not only for ourselves, but for those at the Canteen and the hospital. When a break came, we made a dash for the *cave* next door, but the next day we had mattresses taken to one of the champagne caves and all seventeen of us slept there—at least tried to sleep.

The hospitals were evacuated Saturday, so after that there was nothing more for us to do there and we went back to Canteen work. Saturday night came a telegram from the Ambassador asking the General to make possible Emma's and my return to Paris. Of course, we could not leave like cowards, before the rest of the Unit left, so we sent a telegram to him saying that unless he had bad news for us from home we preferred not to leave—telling him to cable you that we were well and well taken care of. We had an automobile and a *camion*, belonging to the Canteen, and two American Red Cross officers there with big trucks, so we could start at once in something when it was necessary. Of course, one got a little nervous, once in a while, but there was no reason.

Sunday afternoon the first *obus* fell in the town, and that night it was decided that ten of us should leave—seven staying, Emma and I among them, but Monday morning Miss E—— said only the four who could run cars were to stay. Some went to ——, some to ——, and seven of us came here.

We had *musettes* packed for several days ready to leave—expecting two of them were the only things each of us could take, but

177

as we came in a big Red Cross truck, we each brought a suitcase besides. However, most of our things are in two trunks in ———. This is a very quaint, picturesque town with many old buildings. We went to ten places to find a place to stay, and Emma and I are with the widow of a doctor—a quaint house with a lovely garden where I am writing now—the house much run down. We have a very small room for which the lady allows us to pay one *franc* a day. She wished nothing to be paid, as we are working for the French. We take our meals at the hotel—very near. All seven of us are scattered around. A French Canteen is to be opened here and we expect to help in opening it, at least two or three of us. The rest are in the hospitals, and Emma and I helped all yesterday in a French ward, but we are waiting to see in what way and where we will be wanted.

Trains are uncertain, but this letter may reach you, as I hope it will. Don't worry about us, we shall not run into danger, and if it comes to us you don't want us to run away from it, but take it as bravely as other people do. We shall send you word whenever we can. . . .

Lovingly yours

Kate

CHAPTER 3

Letter from Cardinal Luçon

Reims, *le 1ᵉʳ decembre* 1917

Madame,—

Je ne saurais vous dire combien je regrette de ne m'être pas trouvé à la maison quand vous m'avez fait l'honneur de vous y présenter. Il m'eût été très agréable de vous faire visiter notre illustre et chère Cathédrale et de vous expliquer la lamentable histoire des malheurs qui l'ont mise dans l'état où vous l'avez vue. Mon Vicaire Général M. le Chanoine Lecomte a fait ce que je n'ai pu faire moi-même, et il m'a remis la généreuse offrande que vous aviez déposée entre ses mains pour nos malheureux concitoyens de Reims, réduits à la detrésse par l'incendie ou le bombardement de leurs maisons. Je vous en suis infiniment reconnaissant, Madame, et je prie Dieu de vous en récompenser, ainsi qu'en votre dévouement pour nos pauvres soldats blessés ou malades.

Veuillez agréer, Madame, l'hommage de mes respectueux sentiments.

✝ *Sg. Card. Luçon, Arch, de Reims*

Chapter 5

Letter from the Queen's Lady-in-waiting

G. Q. G. Armée beige
20 mai 1918

Chère Mrs. Larz Anderson:—

La Reine me charge de vous remercier bien vivement de la jolie douzaine de mouchoirs brodés que vous lui avez fait envoyer et de celui avec dentelle dont elle a particulierement admire la beauté et la finesse. Votre si aimable attention a bien touché Sa Majesté dont le seul regret est de penser que vous vous êtes donné tant de peines pour Lui procurer cette charmante surprise.

On nous disait dernièrement que vous étiez encore en Angleterre attendant l'autorisation de vous embarquer pour l'Amérique. Nous espérons que vous pourrez bientôt vous reposer dans votre home a Washington de toutes vos fatigues et de votre inlassable dévouement k venir en aide aux pauvres blessés et aux malheureuses victimes de la guerre.

Je joins à ces lignes, chère Madame, deux petites photographies prises par ma cousine lors de la visite que vous avez faite à son hôpital près de Poperinghe. Depuis lors, l'ennemi bombarde tellement cette region qu'elle a été forcée d'evacuer presque tous les baraquements. Elle-même, reste là pour donner les premiers soins aux blessés mais elle est certainement fort exposée. Ma cousine me charge encore de vous dire qu'elle conserve un souvenir reconnaissant de votre visite et du don si bienvenu que vous lui avez fait pour ses ceuvres.

Veuillez, chère Mrs. Larz Anderson, agréer les respectueux hommages de mon mari et être assurée de mes sentiments très sympathiques.

Snoy de Jehay

Chapter 6

This is quoted from a doctor's letter:—

At the base hospitals the wounded arrive by the train load, or in convoys, as the technical expression is. The convoys may follow each other at close intervals, moreover, and the schedules seem to be addicted to the nocturnal habit—trains usually reaching the base sometime in the middle of the night, when the hospital staff is snatching a few hours of rest after utilising all the daylight and adding a few hours at each end in their work in the wards and in the operating rooms.

Following the arrival of a convoy every one works like hell to get them sorted for dressing, operating, etc. The entire hospital looks like a busy day in the dispensary with only one doc present and he having to leave about eleven o'clock—you get me?

Speaking of women's work in war-time Pemberton writes:—

Ruling out heavy mechanical labour, there are few occupations or industries at the Front which women could not serve as well as men. Ask them to drive an ambulance, to become hospital orderlies, to cook, to sew, to make smoke helmets, to keep books, to act as pay mistresses, and in all these employments you will find them capable.

The Green Cross workers are said to do cheerfully the "dirty work," and as they are all women of refinement and intelligence the work is new to them, but there are no slackers. In fact, they have won high commendation for their diligence, and the Standard has respectfully nicknamed them the "Stick-at-Nothings."

CHAPTER 8

Letter from a Nurse at La Panne at the Time the Tea-House was bombed, in April, 1918

You never saw such a place in your life. There is no town left. ...There isn't a window left anywhere and sentries are placed all around to keep the people away for fear of falling glass. ... Strange to say, no one was badly hurt. They had beds and ambulances all ready, but only about five came in, and they had only scratches. ... (*Later*). For the last week we have been getting men in as fast as they could bring them—three hundred a day. We have opened up two new pavilions for gassed men, and have had so many that they have overflowed all over the hospital, besides all the wounded. Extra beds have been put up in every ward, and nurses taken away from us for the new wards and reception ward, so that we have only half the number we usually have and twice the work. We make beds all day long; as soon as a lot come in, those that can be moved are sent to hospitals further back; we sometimes have our beds filled five times a day. We work from eight in the morning until after eight at night without any rest, and we are all looking like wrecks; besides that, they have been bombarding us every night for a week with naval guns. Five of the nurses ... have been killed. ...You

180

have no idea how horrible it has been.

Chapter 9

Extract from a Red Cross Bulletin

The regular pay of the common soldier in the Belgian Army is thirty *centimes* (less than six cents a day), board and keep. When he goes to the firing-line, he gets one *franc* a day—by current exchange, seventeen cents; when he is assigned to a munition factory, he is paid three to four *francs* a day, and if he finds food and lodging for himself, he receives two *francs* extra.

There are several thousand Belgian soldiers who have never had a day of real rest since their mobilisation, for the simple reason that they have no money to spend and no place to go.

They have spent two or three weeks at farm labour in the French countryside, in conjunction with a special service instituted by the Belgian Minister of Agriculture.

Letter from the Countess de Caraman Chimay

Ferme Ste Flore
G^d.Q.G.A.B.
27, 4, 1918

Dear Mrs. Anderson:—

I am desired by the queen to tell you how pleased Her Majesty was to receive your valuable volumes *Odd Corners* with its dedication, and *The Spell of Belgium*.

Her Majesty rejoices herself to read your interesting recollection of happier time in Brussels and I am to convey to you Her best thanks.

Believe me, dear Mrs. Anderson, with kind regards,
Yours very sincerely,
Css. G. DE Caraman Chimay
Lady-in-waiting to H. M. The Queen of the Belgians

Papers in regard to the "Médaille de la Reine Elisabeth"

Moniteur Beige
Journal Officiel
des 23, 24, 25, 26, 27, 28, 29, et 30 septembre 1916
Loi, Arrêtés Royaux et Actes du Gouvernement
Ministère de l'Intérieur
Médaille de la Reine Elisabeth

Sire,—

Le monde entier rend hommage à la charité de la Reine Elisabeth comme à l'honneur chevaleresque du Roi Albert.

Notre Souveraine personnifie la bonté, le dévouement, l'abnégation.

A côte d'Elle et suivant son exemple, nombreuses sont les personnes de toute nationalité et de toute condition, qui sont consacrées dans un esprit de sacrifice, à soulager les affreuses misères de toute nature que la guerre a engendrées.

Votre Majesté reconnait chaque jour, par l'octroi de distinctions honorifiques, les actes d'héroïsmes de nos soldats sur le champ de bataille.

Elle d daigné instituer, par son arrêté du 18 mai 1915, une décoration civique spéciale pour tous ceux qui, à l'occasion des évènements de la guerre, ont, par un acte de courage héroïque, glorieusement manifesté Ieur patriotisme.

Il convient que les nobles dévouements, les sacrifices constants et discrets qui se sont révélés dans les oeuvres de guerre ne tombent pas non plus dans l'oubli et que les personnes chari tables beiges ou étrangères dont ils sont l'honneur, reçoivent un témoignage de la reconnaissance nationale.

Une médaille à laquelle Votre Majesté consentirait à attacher le nom de la Reine Elisabeth, serait pour elles le gage le plus précieux de cette gratitude.

Ce sont ces considérations, SIRE, qui nous ont déterminé à formuler le projet d'arrêté ci-annexé, que nous soumettons respectueusement à la Haute approbation du Roi.

    J'ai l'honneur d'être.

    Sire,

      de Votre Majesté,

           Le très respectueux et fidèle serviteur.
           Le Ministre de l'Intérieur
           Paul Berryer

Le Havre, le 9 septembre 1916

Albert, Roi des Beiges,

    A tous, présents et à venir, Salut.

Voulant honorer les personnes charitables, qui, tant en Belgique qu'à l'étranger, se sont dévouées à soulager les infortunes de toute nature résultant de la guerre.

Sur la proposition de Nos Ministres de l'Intérieur, de la Guerre et de la Justice,

Nous avons arrêté et arrêtons:

Article 1ᵉʳ. Il est institué, sous la dénomination de " Médaille de la Reine Elisabeth," une distinction honorifique destinée à récompenser les personnes beiges ou étrangères qui se sont dévouées aux oeuvres de guerre.

Art. 2. La médaille est en métal blanc, légèrement patiné, de 35 millimetres de diamètre.

A l'avers, elle porte l'effigie de la Reine Elisabeth.

Au revers, une figure de femme, sous les voiles de la nurse, symbolise l'esprit de sacrifice, la soumission à l'oeuvre de devoir et d'humanité, que souligne la devise: Pro Patria, Honore et Caritate.

La médaille est surmontée d'une couronne d'olivier; celle-ci entoure une croix en émaillé rouge lorsqu'elle est destinée à récompenser des dévouements qui se sont manifestés dans les hôpitaux.

Art. 3. Le bijou est suspendu par un anneau à un ruban bleu de soie moirée, avec liséré rose à chaque bord latéral; les bandes du liséré sent larges de 4 millimètres.

La médaille ne peut être detachée du ruban.

Art. 4. Nos Ministres de l'Intérieur, de la Guerre et de la Justice sont chargés, chacun en ce qui le concerne, de l'exécution du present arrêté.

Donné en Notre quartier général, le 15 septembre 1916.

Albert

Par le Roi
Le Ministre de l'Intérieur
Paul Berryer
Le Ministre de la Guerre
Ch. de Broqueville
Le Ministre de la Justice
H. Carton de Wiart

CHAPTER 10

Letter from a Relative of a Soldier in one of the Hospitals at the American Front

Dear Friend:—

A few days ago, I received a letter stating you saw a relative of ours in the hospital at the American front in France. Well, that was a brother of mine, and Father and myself take the liberty to thank you for your kindness in writing to us, stating he was slightly gassed, but was doing nicely, poor boy. But thank God, it was bad enough, but it could have been worse, if the poor boy had been killed. I hope God will grant us that pleasure (*sic*) and bring our dear baby boy to us safe and sound. I have received a few letters from him since he has been in the hospital. He stated he was getting along nicely, but was not discharged from the hospital for duty as yet. He is anxious to get back to his boys again. He also stated he was in a beautiful hospital and was being treated very nicely and getting good care. He said the women folks and the Red Cross nurses certainly were "doing their bit" and that they deserved a lot of credit—that they were wonders. Well, I do not know—Anderson—whether it is "Miss" or "Mrs." or "Mr.," but I thank you for your kindness and hope that someday all the boys will pay you back. Thank you once more for Father and myself.

Letter from a Y.M.C.A. Woman Worker

I am at this most interesting post and simply love the work, as I can see what it means to the boys. We have a very fine type of divisional secretary over us—a Yale man. There are fourteen other secretaries in charge of athletic activities, attending to sending off money, etc., for the boys, entertainment programmes, etc.; every morning they, with the five women workers, have a conference (around the stove, as it is still pretty chilly) and talk over the affairs for the day. It is all rather amusing at times, as these men have a decided sense of humour and we pull together very pleasantly, I must say. The type of man is very fine, and their attractive American faces are very good to see.

The Y.M.C.A. Theatres

In France there are two organisations which are the right and left hands of the American Army, accredited by and working under its control—the Red Cross and the Y.M.C.A. Both are semi-militarised, and the functions of each are assigned by military order:

To avoid duplication of work by the Red Cross and the Y.M.C.A., the following division of activities is prescribed: the Red Cross shall provide for the relief work and the Y.M.C.A, will provide for the amusement and recreation of the troops. Commanding officers will cooperate with the representatives of these two agencies.

In some of the more important camps there are separate auditoriums—except that "auditorium" is altogether too grand a word, for they are just like the other huts, except that there are no tables or canteen, and they are filled with closely packed benches. Sometimes the little stage has a drop-curtain, oftener it hasn't. Once in a while the boys have painted a rudimentary "back drop." It nearly always represents New York Harbour, with the Statue of Liberty. There may be a little gasoline engine coughing its life away outside, and so you may have the luxury of electric lights. Sometimes the light is kerosene lanterns and once in a while candles. But even when there is light enough, it is hard to see, because the place is so filled with cigarette smoke.

The huts are not all so primitive, for in some towns the Y.M.C.A. has taken over regular theatres equipped with stock scenery, where more elaborate plays may be given.

Extract from Red Cross Bulletin

The scheme of life in these French countrysides is very different from that in America. The fields are unfenced; the farmers live in closely built villages of brick or soft stone; the houses stand flush with the street; the barns and stables in walled quadrangles behind, reached by gated wagon-ways. The surrounding fields and roads are intact, except for occasional heavy crops of thistles, and for the shell-holes, dugouts, and trenches which mark the belt where the fighting zone ran. The German commands practiced sabotage on the agricultural implements. In some neighbourhoods they felled orchards in bloom; in others they left them standing. The destruction of the villages was equally irregular, taking place either in the course of fighting, through shell-fire; or, at the time of the retreat, through the systematic wreckage on the part of the German troops by fire, explosions, or the use of rams. In nearly every locality some buildings were left standing susceptible of repair.

The French Government has announced the broad purpose of nationalizing the losses, and as a transitional policy—in addition to the heavy task of clearing away debris and cleaning up sanitary conditions—military and civilian authorities have through the summer been engaged in extensive repair work, contracted for ten thousand portable houses (*maisons démontables*) and erected some hundreds of them.

Twentieth-century French farmers, returning refugees and repatriates have to begin again where North American Indians would begin—by hunting for food, temporary shelter, for clothes to cover them, a few household goods and utensils, such as pots, pans, knives and spoons, and an agricultural implement or two, and perhaps a rabbit and some chickens, and if they are very lucky, a goat or a donkey.

CHAPTER 11

Extracts from Letters from Royalieu by Miss Nora Saltonstall

June 3, 1918.

I would not miss all the experiences that we are having now for anything. It is a satisfactory feeling to see your unit come up to scratch; no complaints, no friction, and none of the endless petty troubles which are always so upsetting when people have the time to think about them. You can picture me as one of the lucky people, who was in a vital spot and was able to help when the push came.

I have been kicking my heels and frothing at the mouth because I am so untrained and can help so little. Of course, it means that those who are experienced are called upon to do everything and work long over time. Mrs. Daly is a wonder, she can work days and nights without stopping; one minute she will be scrubbing the floor of the operating-room, the next talking to a general. No one cares what menial work they do so long as it helps to keep things going.

July 5, 1918.

Three bombs fell on the hospital—killed seven horses and destroyed the material, but no one was hurt.

Mrs. Daly has just been cited for the *Croix de Guerre*. She deserves it because she has worked hard; I believe it is fairly hard for women to get it, so we feel very pleased and proud.

Once having been at the front you cannot bear to be in the second line. You hate to think of all the work to be done and all the suffering and not to be there to try and help out; it always happens that there are never enough people on the spot at the right time and that somewhere else there are a lot more waiting and doing nothing.

Extracts from the Letters of an American Woman in the Belgian Bureau at Berne, Switzerland, written in the Spring of 1918

I have been several times to the trains which brought the children and have seen hundreds of Belgian sick and disabled prisoners come in from Germany on the midnight trains, I was there, too, when the first train of British soldiers arrived. They all seemed so happy to be out of Germany. Everything was most beautifully arranged for them. . . . The English Bureau is wonderfully organised; they send about twenty thousand bread parcels a week and five hundred other parcels a day to their prisoners.

One day we went to the Catholic church, where a *Te Deum* was held for the dead fallen in battle. The church was filled with officers and soldiers *internés* in Switzerland, some ill, others without feet, legs, or arms. The service was very impressive. All of us wept.

M. and Mme. César Thomson, from Brussels, passed through Berne. M. Thomson has been called by King Albert to take charge of a Belgian violin department at the Paris Conservatoire. They have both aged very much since the war began. Their son is still at the Belgian front.

General Leman, the famous Belgian general who has been a prisoner in Germany ever since the fall of the forts of Liège, arrived. One of the rooms at the station was placed at his disposal. Everyone from our Belgian Bureau was there. Many of the Belgian *internés*, too, were in line when the general came into the room, which, of course, was crowded. The Belgian minister read a message from King Albert, to which the general responded; he has an easy flow of speech.

The Swiss are very strict now about letting anything out of the country. Even more than one spool of cotton is not allowed. A Belgian girl who had been in Berne for her health returned to Liège the other day. She had permission to take a few medicines—less than thirty *francs'* worth—but as soon as she reached the German frontier the Huns took every bit away. Oh, no, they didn't pay for it!

Things are getting worse and worse every day. Everything is

gradually giving out. Sugar and milk have been stopped, and tea has gone up; also, soap, so laundry work is expensive. There is, of course, a shortage of coal. . . . It has been the coldest winter in thirty years.

The Huns have built an exposition for industry and inventions on a large vacant space right behind the museum. They are certainly not wasting any time; on all sides they are working out schemes for their commerce after the war. Surely the world won't give them a chance. . . . Someone told me that knowing they will be ostracised, they are already considering plans for starting factories in Switzerland as "*Sociétés Anonymes*," selling their goods as Swiss and putting the money in their own Boche pockets.

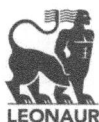

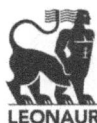